"Fight like the third monkey trying to get on Noah's Ark!"
  - Josh Mercer

THINK
LIKE A
COP

Strategies
to Keep You
and Your Family
Safe

Josh Mercer

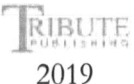

2019

Copyright © 2019
Tribute Publishing, LLC
Frisco, Texas

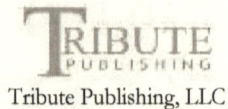

Tribute Publishing, LLC

Think like a Cop
First Edition March 2019

All Worldwide Rights Reserved
ISBN: 978-1-7337727-0-9

All Rights Reserved. No part of this book may be reproduced, stored in a retrieval system, or transmitted, in any form, or by any means, electronic, mechanical, recorded, photocopied, or otherwise, without the prior written permission of the copyright owner or the Author, except by a reviewer who may quote brief passages in a review.

Printed in the United States of America.

In God We Trust.

I would like to thank my family:
Jenny, Parker, Bailey and now Maddie
for their never-ending love and support
in this amazing life adventure.

Table of Contents

My Mission i

Introduction 1

Three Stories of Violence 11

What to Expect 27

Developing Your Black Belt Brain 41

Developing a 360 Awareness 59

Body Language 73

Verbal Jiu-Jitsu and De-Escalation 89

Discovering Your Trouble Bubble 105

Developing a Mental Self Defense 121

Bonus: Top Strategies When Faced with Physical Violence 133

Conclusion 141

About the Author 143

My Mission

My mission is to give you simple tools to keep you and your family safe in today's world without arming you with a weapon or demanding that you take martial arts classes. Self-defense should be simple.

Introduction

You are vulnerable and in danger right now. I am here to help. My mission and my passion is to give you the tools to keep you and your family safe in today's world. My task is to give you the tools to think awareness first, then if violence lands in your lap, the permission to deal with that violence effectively. I want good citizens to be safe.

As a police officer in this day and age, we have had drilled into our heads from the moment we stepped foot in the police academy that we need to keep our heads on a swivel, keep a 360° awareness about us, and keep our defenses up at all times so that we can go home safe to our families after our shift. This is the same awareness that you will need. I have hacked the system and will pass that information on to you.

The TAC Officers that drilled awareness and safety into our skulls for about six months gave their experience and souls to ensure that thirty officers at a time would go home safe at the end of their shifts. Thank you.

Introduction

One day, after a peculiar and exasperating day of chasing bad guys and closer calls than I would care to admit, I got to thinking: "Everyone can own the same kind self-defense and awareness that police officers have, we just have to tell them about it." After sharing some of the concepts with a few individuals who I am close with in my department and other trusted officers, I took the experimental ideas and talked about them in the seminars I was teaching at the time. The idea began to take shape and *Think like a Cop Seminars* was born.

I want to pass a gift on to you in book form. As a patrol officer, I see avoidable violence every day. I am morbidly curious about what leads up to an assault or criminal activity. As a result of my curiosity, I have thrust details of these activities into my tiny mind that I have had a hard time letting loose of because most of them were simply avoidable to begin with.

As a seminar host, I hear horror stories of what is happening to real people who walk real streets and live in real neighborhoods. These streets may be the same ones that you walk. These neighborhoods may be the same ones that you live in. Make no mistake, I don't want violence to be there, but it is there. And if it lands in your lap, I want you to be prepared to not be a victim.

Introduction

I have come to the conclusion that most people are purposely unaware. People are living in the land of unicorns, lollipops, and gumdrops where violence does not exist. These people have created in their mind's eye a utopia that is on the borderline of blindfolded stupidity. Most people refuse to come to some basic self-realization about the world that we live in and the real evil that will befall them if they continue to wander the streets in their utopia bubble.

These are the same people who will turn into a squealing five-year-old if they hear a bump in the night. They pull the covers above their head and ignore the burglar or rapists in the room, thinking that he will just go away. "I can't see you so you can't see me, so now that we have that agreement, after you are finished with me, everything will be OK." WRONG.

Real world people are getting assaulted out of the blue at a staggering rate. According to the FBI, 248.9 out of 100,000 people in 2017 were victims of an aggravated assault. This does not include simple assaults, domestic assaults, etcetera. This does not seem like a high number until you become a statistic and all of a sudden you care because it was you or a loved one who was violently assaulted.

If you would pull your head out of your utopia bubble for a minute, you may be safer. When you realize that there is real violence happening all around you, you may be safer.

Introduction

You may have been lucky and missed it so far. Danger is real, and it is there, lurking in the shadows.

There are usually two types of people who attend my seminars on self-defense and awareness. The first person is the one who has had violence happen to them, and they are not going to take it any longer. This may have been family violence or a random act of street violence, but they know it exists because it has happened to them, and they are done with it. This is usually about forty percent of people who take my class.

The second is the type of person who knows someone who has had unexpected violence in their life and knows it is possible, if nothing else but violence by association. Both types of people acknowledge that there really is no utopia. I applaud them for wanting to change, and I applaud you for wanting to change the way you think about the world.

A real-world example of the non-utopia world we now live in is a game that has been around for a while but is getting stronger. This "game" played by our youth is called "The Knock-Out Game." This game consists of walking up to an unsuspecting person and attempting to knock the person out with one blow. Kids are playing this game. Kids are assaulting businessmen and women and doing real and permanent damage. People have died because they are not aware of their surroundings. Why would this game exist? It is absolutely disgusting!

Introduction

People are afraid to walk down the street for fear of being attacked; that should stop. I became upset and decided to do something about the problem. I started with a program called, "Think like a Cop, Fight like a Girl." We empower women to be aware of their surroundings and fight back like a fierce momma bear if necessary.

If you have flipped on the local or national news channel or glanced through Facebook in the last month, you may have noticed a trend of reporting violence against police officers. If you have paused to listen to a conversation at the gym or overheard a conversation at the grocery store, you will have probably learned about the most recent police officer that was shot, stabbed, ambushed, or killed in the line of duty because of a selfish act of cowardice. We have a dangerous job, and that is why we have to be extremely aware of our surroundings at all times. I want to help pass this awareness on to you.

Because we have a dangerous job, we have developed a superhuman-type skillset that is unique to our profession. It is an amazing skillset that is passed down, taught, and instructed in academies. The only drawback is that it doesn't come with a cape! The skillset is not a secret and it is not held under lock and key. It is a secret that may be hard to describe or hard to translate and put into civilian terms. However, the secret keeps us safe and is practiced both on

Introduction

and off the job with such meticulousness that it becomes second nature, Jason Bourne-ish, if that is a word.

My wife and I were strolling down a public sidewalk hand in hand on a quick little getaway to embrace downtown Portland, Oregon. It was a sunny, glorious morning at about 11:00am when Jenny exclaimed, "You just went into cop mode there, didn't you?" I didn't even realize it, but it seems to happen often enough for us to have a name for it, "Cop Mode." In my mind, Cop Mode also comes with dramatic theme music and a cape, but then again, the kit doesn't come with capes, so my personal view has to be morphed.

I had seen in the distance a disheveled male stumble out from under a cardboard tent. He was hidden in a business doorway a couple of blocks ahead. The male swayed in the swift one-mile-per-hour northwestern breeze. I could see him shouting at the wind and cursing the gods that had placed this blasted cement under his rotten bare feet. He then pulled down his pants to his knees like a five-year-old and urinated in what was going to be our pleasant pathway to VooDoo Doughnut bliss. He swayed around and around as if he was keeping an invisible hula hoop balanced on his hips. The sidewalk was now a river of discarded bad decision juice all in front of God and a courtyard full of men, women, and children. I was indignant and a little entertained because, to be honest, it was kinda funny. Not normal, but funny. I like weird, and we were coming face to face with weird. But

Introduction

I'm not normal, so into cop mode I went. I kept a cool head, switched sides of the street, and put Jenny on the safe side with myself between Mr. Staggering Urination and her.

This happened as a matter of rote practiced forethought. I realized that I didn't really have to think about it at this point, it was second nature. I was not afraid of the magnitude of the steady flow or the blasphemous verbal assault the male had unleashed on his kingdom. There was, however, no reason to be a part of what might have happened or what could be. My reaction to cross the street and place myself between the male and my wife happened automatically because self-preservation and the protection of my family had kicked in way ahead of time. The alert system that I had built into my psyche from the academy days was now working on autopilot.

I realized that I didn't know what this man's intentions were when he rolled from his cardboard condo. I had seen the building blocks of something unusual and out of the ordinary unfolding before Jenny and I had entered a point of no return. I had begun putting my plan together for action ahead of time. Jenny noticed about the time others at the public street fair noticed and began to groan and pick up their phones to take pictures for their Instagram feeds and to call the police to take care of the menace.

I went into Cop Mode ahead of everyone's reaction, about a block and a half away, to be exact. I am not special.

Introduction

This is not something that I picked up with a spider bite or a drop of vampire blood. I cannot leap from building to building in a single bound. I cannot even parkour. This reaction was taught. Hundreds of thousands of police officers across the globe can relate because they were taught by someone who cared for them enough to impart the importance of awareness. I would suggest that is why you picked up this book because now is the time for you to learn.

The academy has taught us about physical self-defense, mental self-defense, and self-preservation. Officers have used this training to the point where it has become a psychological term for overuse. Our 360 Awareness can become a Hypervigilance system put into place to keep us alive whether we are on duty or not. This system, while an effective form of self-preservation, can also be a detriment, making people hyper-aware of their surroundings all the time. Hypervigilance is a distant relative to PTSD. They have locked bloodlines and similar DNA, but could also legally marry if they wanted to.

We do not want to gift you Hypervigilance or PTSD, but something short of that. We want you to be aware of your surroundings and be safe, as well as be able to take care of violence should it land in your lap. Or better yet, avoid it.

Think like a Cop was built so that you could be safe and be your own first responder in a crisis. It was also built so that you can learn to think ahead of time and avoid danger

Introduction

instead of having danger be a surprise. Surprises are great, but violent surprises are not a fun package to receive.

Violence has become a part of our everyday life and social structure. We are, for the most part, immune to it because we see it every day on the news or in the short thirty seconds of the latest Youtube, Instagram, and Facebook liking frenzy. Unless violence or crime strikes us personally, we tend to shrug our shoulders and mutter something to the effect of, "That is something that happened to them." Until "them" becomes personal, and tragedy strikes close to home, we remain at a stiff arm's length from thinking about protecting ourselves or our family.

Police officers see the aftermath of violence every day. Yes, sometimes we are in the middle of a firefight or a gun battle, but for the most part, we are on the outside of the actual act. If we had a crystal ball, we would be there before the act to stop it. There is something built in each police officer that wants to help. We hear the stories of random crime and violence as well as preplanned crimes of selfishness and stupidity.

At the time that violence has already happened, a police officer's advice will fall on deaf ears, and it is largely inappropriate to dispense advice at the scene of a violent act to a victim. It is pandering and sounds like "I told you so." Victims just want the problem solved that is right in front of

Introduction

them. So, when do we have time to dispense quality advise? The answer is usually never.

This book and the seminars we do were built because of the frustration that we cannot be there before an act of criminality happens to you. I want to show you how you can be your own first responder. This is the advice that every law enforcement officer knows and wants to tell you, but may not be able to articulate at the time.

Thank you for picking up this book. I hope to see you at a seminar; it is a fun adult learning environment where you will learn how to become more aware of your surroundings and protect yourselves.

Three Stories of Violence

The following are stories of violence to help you discover what violence is. The way we view violence in our society is usually with scorn and ridicule. However, what if we are the victim and have to use violence to keep us safe? Is that still violence?

STORY NUMBER ONE

Janie was taking groceries out of her car at about four in the morning after her long shift at the hospital. She was getting home about three hours later than she usually did. She had stopped at the grocery store prior to arriving home that night. She really didn't want to get groceries, because after her twelve-hour shift at the hospital she was exhausted. Janie was both mentally and physically drained from the past week and today, the last day of her shift, was crazy busy. This shift seemed to be a special kind of special, a toast to her Friday and to her long week. But it was over, and she could finally relax.

Janie had stopped for a few groceries early this morning because she was feeding all the in-laws for a special surprise dinner. Janie was exhausted but resolved that she would only have time for a make shift nap before meal preparation had to begin for their special night. She knew that her husband was working overtime on top of his normal shift and would be home just in time to shower, change and get ready for the evening. There was no time for him to do the shopping. They usually missed each other on their work days as she worked swing shift and he worked the night shift at the same hospital. It was frustrating, but they made the most of the weekends they had off together. This was a special night because they had the exact same weekend days off, which was unusual. They were looking forward to some time off together before the in-laws arrived, but Jackson got called for an extended shift.

Shift changes were coming in the next few months, and they could finally work on the exact same shift with the exact same hours, but different wings of the hospital. Hopefully, they could even carpool.

Tonight, they were revealing that they were having a baby to all the in-laws. Janie knew that the reveal was going to be special. She was one of eight kids, and this was going to be the first grandchild on both sides of the family. Janie was tired, but giddy with excitement. They had tried for over two years and had finally just given up. Janie and her husband Jackson had sunk their teeth into their work, and they were crawling up the hospital ladder. Things were finally getting easier career-wise, they were relaxed. Then poof! After an extended trip to Mexico, they found out they were pregnant with their first child.

This was going to be an epic surprise. Both sets of in-laws were going to be there for the reveal. They had planned on blue and pink mismatched napkins and other subtle hints, like making a big deal of serving wine and she would not have any. Then, when the dessert arrived, there would be a special announcement on top of the cake, which Janie would have her mother cut and serve. Janie's mother was a squealer, so she and Jackson planned that her mother would be in charge of serving the cake, while the rest of the family would gather around for the pink and blue cake and conversations would commence. She imagined spirited conversations surrounding names, birth dates, boy or girl, and baby shower dates.

Janie had cleared the store where she had picked up the cake and a few last-minute odds and ends. She waltzed out to the car with a skip in her step and a song in her heart; they were finally creating the family they had always dreamed of. She cranked her favorite tunes on the way home and realized after parking in her driveway that her cranky neighbor, Linda, would probably be calling the police again for a noise complaint. *Oh well, I'm worth it!*

Janie unlocked the back hatch to her SUV and pulled out one of the bags of groceries to take into the house. "*I should really take two bags at a time,*" she thought, "*but, I'm pregnant. I'm pregnant!*" she repeated to herself. Janie liked the sound of that! She could hardly wait to announce it. She left the hatch of the SUV up so she could return and gather the remaining groceries.

Janie unlocked the door and danced inside the house to place the first bag of groceries on the kitchen table. She turned and headed back down the hallway to the front door to get the other bag from the SUV.

Janie started to open the front door to go out to her car again and noticed something move in the living room. She thought for a second that Jackson had called in sick for work and was in the living room waiting to surprise her and help with dinner. But it felt weird. The hairs on the back of her neck stood up. She could feel an uneasy chill crawl up her back. Her hand was on the knob, but she glanced back over her shoulder to the living room to say hello to her husband and ruin his surprise.

A strange man was upon her immediately. She turned to face him and push him off, but he shoved her into the door with his body, slamming the door shut. He grabbed her by the hair and yanked her backward. He flipped her around by her neck. They were now face to face. She was staring up at a monster.

The man was large and rough; he had long, oily hair and a three-day-old scruff. The man had crooked teeth, and his breath smelled horrible as he thrust himself in her space. She remembered he was breathing heavy and had a guttural sound when he breathed in her face. He put his hands around her throat and flung her against the hallway wall.

He didn't say anything.

The action almost knocked the wind out of Janie. She struggled for breath and balanced on the tips of her toes while she struggled to get free from the wall and his hands wrapped around her throat. She gasped for another breath with a big gulp. She flailed.

"Why?" She managed to finally get out. "Why!?"

She felt his grip tighten; he grunted as he strained to squeeze her neck. She could see her attacker squint his eyes, but there was no other emotion on his face. Except for his breathing, he was silent.

"What are you doing?" Janie got out. "Why!? Stop!" She gurgled.

Janie's back was tight against the wall. All she could think of was "*WHY?*" She tried to scream, but all that came out was a gurgle and sputter against his gigantic, rough, monster hands. He grunted some more in anger and frustration that she was not lifeless yet. He lifted her up higher, so she could not balance on her toes any longer. He squeezed her neck and growled angrily. She placed both her tiny hands on his oversized meat hooks and attempted to pry them away. She scratched and hit at his hands and arms; it was no use. She tried to reach his face, but her arms were too short. Janie wiggled and thrashed about, squeaking and gasping for air. Things began to tingle, then everything went black.

When she woke up, the police and medics were standing beside her. There was blood everywhere. Janie could not feel the left side of her face. She asked to see a mirror and the medics would not let her. Janie knew that was a bad sign. She felt her face, it was swollen and raw on the left side. She asked where all the blood came from and the medics told her that she was assaulted. She could not remember what had happened. Then, parts slowly came back to her.

She collapsed after she was choked but woke up as he had kicked her in the head. She had woken up again during the assault to see a fist coming down to meet her eyeball. She blacked out again. She remembered not being able to see, but feeling the forceful blow after blow to her face as she went in and out of consciousness.

At the hospital, she found out that she had been violently assaulted, raped, and left for dead. She lost the baby. She spent months in rehabilitative and reconstruction surgery for her face, and years later still had flashbacks from the event.

The neighbor lady had indeed called the police for a noise complaint. She told the police that there was some violent music playing and it was well past the noise ordinance of ten o'clock for the city. Linda demanded that something be done about the vile nuisance next door.

Once the police got there and saw the open trunk of the SUV, they investigated further. When they looked through the window, they found the bloody scene by the front door.

She later explained to the police that she had left the door open for a second while she was unloading groceries. The man must have slipped in the door without her knowing about it and attacked her. She must have surprised him at the front door when she went back for the second round of groceries.

STORY NUMBER TWO

Janie had cleared the store and waltzed out to the car with a skip in her step and a song in her heart; they were finally creating the family they had always dreamed of. She cranked her favorite tunes on the way home and realized after parking that her cranky neighbor, Linda, would probably be calling the police again for a noise complaint. *Oh well, I'm worth it!*

Janie unlocked the back hatch to her SUV and pulled out one of the bags of groceries to take into the house. *"I should really take two bags at a time,"* she thought *"But I'm pregnant. I'm pregnant!"* she repeated to herself. Janie liked the sound of that! She could hardly wait to announce it.

She placed the first bag of groceries on the kitchen table and quickly moved down the hall to retrieve the other bag from the SUV.

Three Stories of Violence

She started to open the front door to go out to the car again and noticed something move in the living room. She thought Jackson had called in sick for work or something and was in the living room. But it felt weird. The hairs on the back of her neck stood up. She glanced back in the living room, and a strange man was upon her immediately.

The man was large and rough. He had a three-day-old scruff. Crooked, unbrushed teeth snarled at her as he barreled in toward her; his breath smelled horrible! He pushed himself against her, violating her private space. He put his hands around her throat and thrust her against the far wall in the hallway.

The attacker didn't say anything. He just grunted. Janie was caught off guard for a second, was this happening? She gathered her bearings. The force almost knocked the wind out of her. She took a deep breath as the realization came over her that this was a life or death situation and it was happening to her right now. There was no time to call the cops. There was no time to scream, nobody would hear. There was no time to do anything but fight for her life, and the life of her unborn child.

Janie felt the man's rough sandpaper hands begin to tighten around her neck as he grunted, still not saying a word. He grunted and pressed harder, lifting her up against the wall.

Three Stories of Violence

Janie knew that if both her attacker's hands were around her neck that other areas of his body were exposed. She knew that her attacker was bigger and stronger than she was. She knew that she would have to use all of her power, strength, and might to subdue this monster and get away. It was him or her. Life or death. Right Now!

She knew she had to meet violence with brutal, excessive violence in order to survive. She made the decision to fight and fight with all her willpower, all her power, and all of her strength. This was an easy decision because she had already made it a month before when she found out she was pregnant; she was going to protect her child with her life. She could feel her eyes begin to blur on either side of her vision as a black tunnel began to form. She was going to pass out and it would be over.

Janie placed both of her tiny feet on the wall behind her and her hands on her attackers strong harry knuckles that were wrapped around her throat. She pushed against the wall with all her might. She kicked him right in the solar plexus. He grunted loudly but did not let go. She kicked him again as hard as she could; his grip loosened as his hands began to sink toward his mid-section. Janie braced herself against the wall as her vision began to clear. She gave the intruder one final kick as hard as she could, penetrating her attacker up the center of his body, through his groin, and up into his diaphragm as if her shin was a Samurai sword and she was cutting him in half from the bottom up. She thought she lifted him off of the ground with her tiny leg.

He began to bend over slightly in pain. The attacker had paused his attack on Janie as he buckled forward slightly. She then clasped her hands around his neck and thrust up with her right knee while bringing his neck and head downward as hard as she could. She felt the pop of his nose and a spurt of warm liquid hit her in the arm. Her attacker now was doubled over and backpedaling to get away from this tiny devil. He hit the end table and stumbled backward, knocking over the lamp and several knickknacks. She had time and space now; she could get away.

Janie ran out of the open door of her house. Realizing that she had left her keys in the house, she ran to her cranky neighbors. Linda was already on the phone with the police reporting the loud music that was shaking her windows this late at night. Linda had not realized that there was an assault happening next door, but when she saw Janie spring from the doorway scared and disheveled, she knew something was wrong. She opened her door and called for Janie to take refuge in her house. Janie was finally able to scream for help. She was bloody from the assault. Linda welcomed her with open arms and quickly shut the door behind her.

Janie blurted out. "I'm pregnant!" She immediately regretted saying that to Mrs. Grumpy Pants, but nothing else came out at first. Eventually, she was able to articulate to

Linda about the assault and Linda relayed it to the police dispatcher.

Within minutes the police got there. The attacker had fled the scene. They did a K9 track and found the male hiding in a bush about a block away. He was unable to run far due to his injuries of blunt force to the groin, and he could not see well because of his exploded nose. Sgt. Smith told Janie later that her attacker had several felony warrants for a recent kidnapping and rape. He went to the hospital and then to jail for this third felony strike. He would not get out for a while.

Janie was checked at the hospital. She had no permanent injuries. She kept the baby.

STORY NUMBER THREE

Janie had cleared the store and waltzed out to the car with a skip in her step and a song in her heart; they were finally creating the family they had always dreamed of. She cranked her favorite tunes on the way home, singing and dancing in the car.

About two blocks away she remembered that her cranky neighbor, Linda, would probably have a conniption fit about the loud music. *Oh well, I'm worth it!* She turned the music off and thought, *Why stir up trouble? This is going to be a family neighborhood now. Maybe Linda could be converted to a nice person? We will save that for another day.*

Three Stories of Violence

Janie rolled her window down slightly to catch some fresh, fall air as she coasted quietly up the block to her house. She noted that something felt different as she drove up. There was a slight movement by the tree. The shadow was moving. Weird! The tree stood about ten feet from the sidewalk into Janie's yard. She thought about how the mature tree would soon hold a tire swing and laughter from her new family. *How dare the shadows move and scare me like that!* She attempted to play it off like that for a moment, but then realized that the shadow was actually moving, and it was not part of the tree.

To the side of the house, walking along the sidewalk, was a man who didn't belong. He was tall and disheveled; he looked out of place in their neighborhood. It seemed as though he had just stepped out from behind the tree that was in Janie's yard. *I wonder if he was urinating on my property!? How RUDE!* She didn't want to judge anyone, but this guy was giving her the creeps! This was the kind of person that would be downtown begging for money, not out in the suburbs. Something was wrong. Why was he here?

As Janie coasted quietly into the circular driveway, she looked into the driver's side mirror and noted that the male who had been walking away from her had suddenly turned and was now facing the house.

The stranger was now attempting to hide behind a hedge at the far end of the driveway. He was lurking from the sidewalk. This made Janie feel uneasy. He didn't know she could see him in the driver's side mirror, but she could. He had crouched down a bit and attempted to conceal himself in the shadows the street lights cast against the trees in the neighborhood.

Janie got a strange feeling that crawled up her spine. This isn't right! This really isn't right! I am NOT getting out of the car here. No way! She drove off while calling the police, reporting that there was a strange man lurking in the bushes in the neighborhood. Janie told the police dispatcher what she saw, and a brief description of the male.

About an hour later, Sgt. Smith called Janie. We caught the man who was in your neighborhood. The man had several outstanding felony warrants for his arrest, including burglary, kidnapping, and rape. Smith advised that he had gotten dropped off in the area after being let out of prison a few short months ago. He was going to see his mother and was hoping to hide from the law just a few blocks away. His mother had kicked him out of the house due to his violent behavior and did not want anything to do with him. Smith thanked Janie for the call. She told Sgt. Smith that something about him just creeped her out!

Sgt. Smith assured Janie that he would be going back to prison for his recent crime spree and she would not have to worry about him creeping in the neighborhood again.

Three Stories of Violence

Of the three stories, two were violent, and one was observant awareness. Which would you rather choose? I know, dumb question when you know the outcomes. However, most people will ignore the potential for violence and choose to live in oblivion. You are not most people and are making changes to your awareness right now. Good job.

In the first two stories of violence, we could clearly identify with the hero of the story and would pat her on the back if we were to hear the second story in person. However, the story is violent nonetheless. What makes it different? Our morals, values, societal rules? Yes, all of those.

The three stories are, of course, fictional, however not far off from the day-to-day activities of the criminal mind in every city worldwide. The stories illustrate a few points:

Violence is violence. There is unjustifiable violence as in the case with the first story. Everyone who reads story number one wants to take the assailant out behind the woodshed and do unspeakable things to him. This is the bad type of violence, and we as a society do not put up with it. It is unacceptable.

Then there is justifiable violence, as in the case with the second story. Everyone who reads story number two wants to pat this lady on the back and give her a spot on the national news to tell her story because of her heroic actions. This is justifiable violence. But it is still a violent act. The roles just got reversed, and Janie took on a violent roll. And we applaud her for it.

Awareness. There is no hero's parade for awareness. There are no national spots on the news for a random act of awareness. There should be, but there isn't. Awareness means that we get to avoid violence ahead of time, or not get to the point of violence at all. It is not as impressive of a story, but you will always live to tell the tale of walking away rather than taking a chance at being like the number one story and placed in the FBI statistics journal.

You have a choice. You can choose to be unaware and oblivious to what is around you all the time and take the chance that you may encounter violence by surprise. Or you can choose to become aware of your surroundings and avoiding violence altogether. The second part to that choice is that if violence is put in your lap and you have to deal with it, then *fight like you are the third monkey trying to get on Noah's Ark!* Give violence back to your attacker with all you have for the protection of yourself and for your family.

As a police officer, I often see that people chose to be a victim (as in story number one) because they have never given themselves permission to fight violence with violence for their own safety. No, they did not choose to be put in a situation with a violent outcome. They did not ask to be assaulted, but sometimes they choose to not fight back because they have not given themselves permission to do so.

Three Stories of Violence

Society has taught us to be nice all the time; even when we may not survive, we have to be polite. Not so. It is a choice. You may have to choose someday to save the life of your family and your own life. I hope you choose you!

I am giving you this choice now so that you can know what to expect on the other side of violence. So that you can choose now to be a survivor. Pick you. You are worth it.

What to Expect

Daryl was shopping in a good neighborhood on a peaceful, tranquil Sunday afternoon. He was in a rather upscale outlet mall with clean streets and burly security guards that patrolled the area. He imagined that they were police officers hired for an off-duty gig to help the customers feel all warm and cozy. There was never a real threat in this area that he knew of. The local news had to borrow violent news from other counties just to fill the violent quota and keep sales of the paper up. This was a good neighborhood with good people. The stores that surrounded the mall were ones that attracted good people and didn't put up with riff-raff.

Daryl noted that the security guys looked bored as they dispensed directions to bathrooms and unlocked a nice older Mercedes for an elderly blue hair that had the misfortune to leave her purse in her front seat with her keys conveniently tied to the strap of the purse.

Daryl only had pants to pick up. He had pre-selected them on a previous trip so he was sure to be in and out of the store in short order. A perfect shopping trip for Daryl.

What to Expect

He hated crowds and hated shopping. He had planned the trip for the end of the shopping day for just this reason. No people, no lines, no parking hassle. This was easy.

Daryl finished his shopping quickly and exited the store with his new purchase. He never thought he would spend one hundred and fifty-seven dollars for jeans, but his wife said he looked amazing in them, so what was he going to do? Disappoint her? NO! He was going to look smashing for their date tonight. Besides, the kids didn't need college anyway; they could go to community college and work at Lawns-n-More just like he did when he was struggling through college. He got a good workout and learned a few words of practical Spanish.

The surrounding stores were closing for the day. He recalled the slow grinding sound of the roll down doors as they began to rumble closed on either side of him as he stepped off of the curb and headed to his car about thirty paces away. He was parked directly across from the store and next to a light post. It was winter, so it was dark at about five o'clock as he stepped from the curb.

Daryl could immediately tell something was going to happen, something was wrong. He knew it somehow. The hair on the back of his neck stood up, and he could feel a pressure, a queasy feeling in his gut. Daryl said his vision began to narrow and focus, but he could not tell why. He began to look around from left to right. The lot was fairly empty of cars, except for what must have been some employee cars sprinkled in the mall parking lot. Daryl said that he was probably the last person in the mall this late. There were no obstructions other than the random vehicles and a few low bushes along the back part of the lot. He felt almost queasy, something was startling, and he couldn't pinpoint it. He did not feel alone in the parking lot.

A figure then appeared out of the shadows at a short distance to his right. He could pinpoint the feeling now; it was associated with the sound of a man's shoe scraping on the ground. The sound was more of a flopping and grinding on the pavement as he limped out of a shadow that the security light had cast on a vehicle parked by a neighboring store. It didn't look like the male was trying to hide in the shadow, but just appeared out of it and was walking toward him.

As Daryl headed for his vehicle at a faster pace, the large white male in his early twenties with a scraggly blond beard, ruffled clothes, and ripped jeans, closed in on him quickly. The male was dirty and mangled somehow. He walked aggressively toward Daryl's direction. The male was far enough away when Daryl first saw him, but he was closing the distance too quickly for comfort.

Closing the distance this quickly added to Daryl's anxiety in the situation and captured additional undue attention. Daryl said, "The guy looked into my eyes. He was locked on, but his soul was missing. Something in his eyes said he didn't care." Daryl said, "The guy was looking right at me, but through me at the same time somehow... it was really weird!"

Daryl acknowledged him by putting up his hand in a "stop" type of motion. He indicated he did not need anything the stranger was selling, giving, or asking for. Daryl said he could see the guys hands, clenching and unclenching. He was breathing heavy and talking to himself. Daryl said that he might have been talking to him, but it was like he was talking himself into something. It was a low, guttural noise that added to Daryl's anxiety in the matter. Daryl recognized later that the male was clenching his teeth in an almost grinding motion. His jaw was chiseled, and the muscles were clenching and unclenching like he was chewing gum without the gum. The man's face was unshaven yet had marks like large raisin-sized razor burns on most of his face.

Based on Daryl's training and experience, he estimated this oncoming writhing mess was probably meth-induced, but he recalled the smell of alcohol in his later dissertation to the police.

Daryl was in the healthcare field and had seen plenty of this kind of behavior, only in a controlled hospital-type environment. Daryl had also spent some time in the inner city as a medic and knew that what was coming at him was drug-induced and probably at the peak of his high. There was no telling what this guy wanted.

The male started angling toward Daryl with his left hand out and asking for something. He seemed almost zombie-like. Daryl was trapped; he was too far to get to his car, and if he turned around his back would be exposed to an unknown threat. He also knew that the doors were closing behind him. But the stranger was advancing so quickly. He didn't want to take his eyes off of him for fear of losing precious seconds for a look at a possible safety net that he knew might not actually be an option.

He felt alone and trapped by the meth zombie aggressively approaching him. Daryl decided to hit the problem straight on. Daryl enlarged his chest and took a wide defensive stance on the balls of his feet. He raised his hands in front of him with his palms out to indicate that he didn't want any part of this nonsense and to protect his vital organs in case things went sideways.

The male's hand was shaking bad, he couldn't keep it still. It was like he had uncontrollable hand and arm tremors. The male said, "You better give me your... your... or... I'll hurt you! I'll cut you REAL BAD!" The male's teeth remained closed as he clenched his demand. Daryl said that the male stammered, stuttered, and twitched so badly that he was not exactly sure what was said, but it was evident that it was a threat and was without a doubt directed toward him because

What to Expect

there was nobody else in the parking lot. Daryl was just about to tell the man to go pound sand and to get away from him when the stranger reached around his back with his right hand. They were about ten feet apart now, and the stranger was still advancing uncomfortably fast.

Daryl did not know what the stranger's intentions were with his right hand; was it a knife, gun, rock, hammer, a bag of gummy bears? He hoped it was gummy bears, gummy bears are delicious! Then he saw it... just the butt end tip of what he knew to be a knife. A black object began to emerge from the male's side pocket of his pants, or maybe it was a holster, he didn't know, it was just bad and it was not going to be gummy bears! He was disappointed.

Daryl told me later that the whole time frame to this point took about three to five seconds. He had time to react but did not have time to think. This was not a proactive, step-back-and-call-the-police moment. This was a fight for his life. The threat was coming to him quickly and the man was demanding and threatening loudly that he was going to hurt Daryl really badly if he didn't get what he wanted, whatever that was.

Daryl's family flashed in his mind, and he was determined to make it out of this.

What Daryl DID know was that it was clearly an immediate physical threat. He felt intimidated, trapped, threatened with his life, and he didn't know yet what the male wanted. Was it his money, the new pants he just purchased, or his life? Daryl only knew this was NOT going to end well if he didn't do something to protect himself.

Daryl calmed himself and picked his target. He stepped in and struck first with brutal violence, hard, and through the intended target: the attacker's knee, about a quarter inch up. He hit the knee with his shin as hard as he could. Daryl described the crack and release like a large twig snapping over your shin before putting it on a campfire. The male went down hard on the cement and smashed his head on the concrete. He was out. The fight and the violence were over for him.

When the male woke up, he puked because he was in so much pain. The aggressor had been running on so much adrenaline, drugs, and alcohol that were pulsing through his body, it was too much for his body to handle. The aggressor could not physically run or walk away, and he could not fight. He was disabled at the scene.

At this point, a store employee who had seen the action unfolding had alerted other store employees. She had called the police, and she and the other employees helped contain the felon at the scene until police arrived.

Total time on the security video for the attack was about four seconds. The self-defense moment was about .75 seconds of that. Most of the .75 seconds of time was the aggressor falling to the ground and hitting his head on the pavement.

Daryl and the police officers later found a large black Bowie type knife ten feet away that had slid from his attacker's grip and scooted under his car. The knife had dried blood on it. The police only speculated that it was from another attack, but could not find any other victims at the time in the vicinity.

The ambulance took the male to the hospital then the police took him to jail. Daryl spent some time talking with the police and giving a written explanation of what had happened. He also said that he spoke with detectives later, which confirmed that he had dealt with a career criminal who was known two counties over for robbing people at knifepoint to get his next high. The male had two outstanding warrants for robbery with a deadly weapon. It could have been worse, right?

Daryl made it to his date with his wife, and he had a story to tell.

What if that was you?

The realities of coming under this kind of pressure, even for a few seconds in your life, can have devastating effects lasting for the rest of your life if you do not have a process. The process will not only give you the confidence to feel safer on the street, but at your job, at your business, or even

What to Expect

at the mall or at a church where you may have to confront the violence that finds you out of the shadows.

I want you to be safe. That is why I do what I do.

In this book and the seminars, I show you how to *Think like a Cop* so that you can be safe and protect yourself and your families. I want you to feel like you can use this thinking anywhere and at any time to heighten your sense of awareness and danger, like a Jedi Master with a hankering for doughnuts and coffee.

To accomplish this, we will develop your Black Belt Brain, your body language, your verbal skills, and your de-escalation skills. I want you to learn about developing your comfort zone that we call your Trouble Bubble, an area of personal awareness and safety that is your own space. In the process we will discuss some of the magic sauce that police officers use both on and off duty to enhance their safety. These skills are easy to learn and practice, and they will, when implemented, keep you safer.

We will break down the body language of a police officer and what it says to a bad guy or criminal. We will give you some tips about how to present yourself like a confident police officer who has had years on the job. These are the same things new police officers learn over several years of on the job experience. Take our experiences and make them your own to keep you and your family safe.

What to Expect

We will learn some new verbal skills that will enable you to thwart off bad guys with just your mouth. This is not to say that if you run your mouth, you will be safe. It is what and how you say things, along with how you stand and present yourself using your newfound body language, that will keep you out of an altercation and will hopefully keep you safe. It is as much what you don't say sometimes as what you do say to show your would-be attackers that you are a hard target, and they may just decide to pick on someone else.

Lastly, you will learn in the bonus chapter some physical elements needed in a violent conflict, should one arise. These techniques are easy to remember, and in our seminars, we will have you physically practice them at full speed on a live person in a protective suit. Super fun! See the back pages of the book for my website and contact information.

The process of becoming a police officer is a long and arduous process; I am about to short-circuit the process of awareness and self-protection for you and share with you some thin blue line secrets.

Police officers train for awareness and self-defense. We learn by someone passing down information that works. We learn by experience what to say and how to say it to the most hardened criminals. These criminals will lie, cheat, and steal from their grandmothers for their next fix. Police officers train as if their lives depend on it (because it does) for about

What to Expect

six months in the basic academy. This gives them the basic knowledge, but only the basics. The basic academy is a canned environment with pretend criminals, false stories, and make-believe scenarios. The graduates have still never tested their newfound skills on a real bad guy. They then enter into the real-world streets and train with hardened, salty professionals who know the ropes of the job.

It is this knowledge that is condensed down to relatable, civilian content that is easy to learn and apply to your everyday life.

At the end of this book, you will have the ability to:

- Develop your Black Belt Brain further. This is no guarantee that you will be able to move like a ninja, strike like an MMA warrior, or think strategically like a master chess player, but you will be closer.
- Develop and put into practice a natural 360-degree awareness of your surroundings.
- Develop your own personal, powerful, authoritative stance and body language.
- Hone and develop a verbal Jiu-Jitsu skillset that will allow you to de-escalate a potential attack quickly.
- Lastly, we will suggest for you to develop a mental self-defense to help you withstand any mental violence or anguish that this world can throw your way.

What to Expect

The information in this book comes from a police officer's desire to help. I became a police officer to be proactive and get involved in the community, only to find that it is really a reactive job. I get a call and react to it, I get another call and react to it. I know people think we sit in a coffee shop eating doughnuts and waiting for our crystal ball to glow blue. The crystal ball will then guide us to the next crime that is afoot, but that is simply not the case. Sometimes we get to bring people to justice on the spot, but most times we take calls that are reactionary at best.

I have researched and have certifications in Neuro-Linguistic Programming. I study body language. I am morbidly curious about physical altercations. I work and live with the science of reading people because my job and my life depend on it. I have taught people how to stand, talk, and fight with an unfair advantage. I am curious about actions and reactions to violence prior to and during altercations. I don't think there is a degree in that. If there was, there would probably be math involved. Yuck! So far it is the school of hard knocks for me, and I am working on my Ph.D.

I have personal, intimate experiences with violence, having been raised in a violent environment. As a result, I don't like bullies! Because I have had an unhealthy prior relationship with violence, I understand what it takes to avoid it or deal with it. Either is fine with me, but it is safer to avoid it if you can.

What to Expect

Developing Your Black Belt Brain

Martial artists can spend many years performing and perfecting their art to earn a black belt. The typical karate black belt can be earned in about five years of hard work and dedication. Judo, Aikido, Kung Fu, and Taekwondo all have similar time frames of commitment while Brazilian Jiu-Jitsu can take ten to twelve years of commitment and have varying degrees of competition within the different disciplines of Jiu-Jitsu.

Becoming a black belt is hard, I don't care what discipline you are in. I do not want to minimize anyone's efforts. Getting into the ring with a practiced Jiu-Jitsu practitioner for a sporting event would be a short, foolish errand. However, in the street, practical applications are not a sporting event. This is violence and it is different. A martial artist practitioner may have an edge in a street fight but practicing in a dojo is vastly different from the rules on the street. Even martial arts have rules where we practice NOT hurting each other in order to keep practicing. Otherwise we would run out of partners quickly.

What I want to stress to you is that you do not need to be a black belt to protect yourself in a bad situation. What you do need to do is wrap your mind around the idea that violence can happen to you without notice and without provocation; it is a surprise and can happen in an instant.

This surprise violent attack can happen while you are walking down the street, while you are on the bus, train, or sitting in traffic. Violence can happen at any time and at any place. It's like a surprise gift from your gran-gran of a hand knitted, bunny-eared sweater when you are twenty-six and graduating law school. It is just plain unwanted, yet for a short time you have to own it, it is your obligation.

You need to prepare your mind first before you need to use your body to protect yourself. You need to be OK with flipping the script from walking around with a victim mentality to walking with confidence that you can take care of yourself.

At the moment of violence, you need to have already given yourself permission to destroy an attacker if necessary. You will know ahead of time because you have planned to do what you know you need to do to be safe and get away. If violence is forced on you, you need to own the mentality that will turn the tables and make the aggressor the victim. You need to own the fact that you can and will be able to hurt someone else to keep yourself and your family safe.

Developing Your Black Belt Brain

Mark Twain said that, "It is not the size of the dog in the fight, but the size of the fight in the dog," which I take to mean it is not the size of the aggressor, but the willingness to survive by the victim in a violent altercation that will determine the outcome. It is the mental edge, the psychological attitude, and your own personal "why" you have given yourself to survive that will give you the mental edge to fight with all it takes to survive and live to see another day.

Make no mistake about it, you are vulnerable, and you are in danger in this day and age without this attitude of survival. You need to give yourself the permission right now to survive. If you can do that, you have a chance.

I can give you the tools of the trade to Think like a Cop. I can give you a unique way to practice and give you a spark to light your awareness bonfire, but unless they are put into effect in your mind, the tools will be rendered useless on the street and in your heart because you will still have a victim mindset that you don't want to hurt someone. You must and need to set your mind free to know beyond a shadow of a doubt that you can and will take down any enemy that brings violence to you.

If you are not willing to do damage to a guy who is trying to do horrible things to you or take your life, then we are done before we start.

Developing Your Black Belt Brain

Only you can affect you. Your willingness to accept new ideas and your willingness to expand your thoughts were demonstrated by picking up this book or attending a seminar. It would suggest that you are there and ready to learn. You are ready to accept the challenge that you may need to hurt someone to be safe if violence finds you.

I was doing a seminar called *Think like a Cop, Fight like a Girl* in Washington State for a group of ladies of mixed ages.

I got to the physical portion where we started to talk about what to do if violence comes to you.

While describing the method in which to gouge an eye of an attacker, I explained that if given the opportunity, take it. If an attacker cannot see you, they cannot chase you, and if they are in pain, they may also forget about attacking you because they are more focused on their own pain. Use this opportunity to get away.

The woman's group that I was speaking with gasped, to my delight, in disgust at the idea of gouging an eye. I went into detail about what it would feel like and what it would look like for them. I went on to hand out grapes and had them squish them in between their thumb and forefinger emulating the crunch and squish of the eyeball in an eye socket as you pop it inward. It is a very tactile description because reality training and shock adult learning are the things that stick with you far beyond going to a seminar, sitting in a seat, taking notes, and coming out with a couple of ideas written on paper. In short, reality training is better and more memorable.

In this case, I may have gotten a little carried away with the description, but it was important, and I really wanted them to get the point. The noises of the group began to amplify. Some of the younger crowd began to put their hands over their mouths. I stopped short of anyone having to use the garbage can or run for the bathroom. I think they got the point.

I could see that one older participant was a little distraught, but didn't seem like she could formulate a sentence at the time. We finished the demonstration of how to find the eyeballs if you needed to. You find the top of the head and grasp it with both hands, then place your thumbs on the forehead and slowly slide your thumbs down over the eyebrows and into the eye sockets. The thumbs fit nicely there. And from there you can squeeze effortlessly inward toward the attacker's eyes and something should pop.

I could tell that the older participant was stumped for a few moments. She had a question, but couldn't articulate it out loud. Finally, she raised her hand and asked the best question ever, "What if I hurt the guy and it causes permanent damage?"

I was proud of her for stepping up with that question because I know that most people have the exact same reaction as she did to hurting someone. The difference was that she was brave enough to ask the question that was on everybody else's mind.

It can be devastating to your psyche just thinking about hurting someone else, let alone planning on it and practicing for it. We had talked about the squeeze, the pop, and most likely the squish and the liquid that would result in the pressure of forcing an eyeball into the socket. We talked about the damage that it would do to the attacker. But we hadn't yet talked about what is affected in the psyche of the person who does this kind of damage to someone else, a real living and breathing person.

I always just assumed that if someone was going to do harm to me that he is fair game and knew that this was not going to end well for him. Maybe you are the same, or maybe you need to give yourself permission ahead of time to hurt someone else so that you and your family are safe. If you had never thought about it, now is the time.

This was a nice, gentle lady who I would imagine went to the corner church every Sunday and had Bible study on Wednesdays from noon to two in the afternoon. She spent her time doing things for others and not thinking about taking care of herself. She probably made cookies for the bake sale to send little Joey and Theresa to summer camp. I imagine that she also bought cookies from the Girl Scouts when they knocked on her door. She was a good person, she was an amazing woman. She had little to no thoughts about things that could happen once she got out of the locked doors of her church, the comfort of her home, or the crowds at the grocery store. She probably never thought that there could be a rapist hiding behind a bush to push her in his waiting car after church Bible study next Wednesday afternoon and drive her to his cabin in the woods for a retreat with the devil.

Sorry to burst your bubble, but these things happen, and the sooner you prepare your mind for this reality, the safer you will be. If you have never thought about bad possibilities before, you have not prepared.

I explained to the nice lady and the group that the person who is going to attack you is not your friend, he is not an acquaintance, and he is not someone who you would invite to lunch on a bright and sunny day to have crumpets and tea in your backyard. This is a person who has brought violence to you and wants to do you harm. Your attacker may just want your wallet, but he does not care about you and he is willing to do serious, devastating harm in the form of violence to get it.

He, in most cases, has pre-planned this attack to pick you out and do damage to you for little or no reason but to get those delicious home-baked cookies because he is hungry. He does not understand that if he asked you for the cookies that you may even give him one or 12. He may be a bully and take with violence because that is what he does. He may yank your arm so hard trying to get that purse off of your shoulder that it pops your shoulder out of your socket, causing months of rehabilitation, doctor visits, x-rays, lost work, and psychological trauma. He resorts to violence because he needs a heroin fix or he will be sick. He can turn in your iPhone at the mall for fifty dollars quick cash without going to the pawn shop and talking to Guido. He knows Guido will take his identification and the police can track who did this crime. His reasons could be to just be a bully, take your money, or in worst cases, kidnap you, stuff you in a trunk, and do unspeakable things to you over the course of several years while you are chained to a concrete bedpost.

In most cases, we may not be able to understand why. In fact, why they bring violence to you doesn't matter. We may want the answer to why someone is trying to hurt you, but we will never get it. It is just violence for violence sake, and it is unacceptable.

If you think that this is just a "stranger danger" problem, then you are dead wrong; this can happen with someone you know. You need to be OK with having the mental capacity to be a whistleblower and stand your ground. That person you know that is a bully is not your friend, relative, acquaintance, or someone you want to have in your life either.

Regardless if your attacker knows you or doesn't, the same idiom applies: He/She is not your friend and never will be. Stop him/her in their tracks before they do damage to you or others.

Also, if you think that victims of violence are just a female problem, then you would be wrong as well. Most reported incidents are from females because males are too macho to admit that they got taken or hurt, but make no mistake, the problem is universal, random, and gender neutral.

You should feel an obligation to send the aggressor to the hospital and then jail with a permanent reminder that it is not OK to pick on people. You are also preventing and stopping the violence that will happen to someone else down the road. You have to mentally prepare for that moment. If that moment never comes, great, at least you are prepared.

As I explained this concept to the women in the seminar, lightbulbs began to fire in the room, and they got empowered. It is not about just them; it is about every potential attack that this person could do on others in their lifetime. They took ownership of the moment and rocked the rest of the class. They will not go willingly. There will be a fight if violence comes to them. They will be safe.

The lady who was brave enough to ask the question from the class was also empowered with that knowledge and went on to excel in the class. Crushing it, in fact. She gave herself permission on the spot to do damage where damage was necessary for her to be safe.

Later, I had a private conversation with her. She has a reason to live. She has grandkids, she has daughters and a son who still need her. She has a husband that she loves, two dogs, and a cat that need her. She made a commitment at that moment that a person who brings violence to her is not deserving of her respect, her love, or her friendship. She made the decision that she did not have to be friends with everyone, and if the moment came, she would be able to act without conscience to put down her attacker so that she could live for her why.

I went back to her original question, "What if you hurt the guy and it causes permanent damage?" She simply said, "Well, I guess he will have a nice little reminder not to be a criminal." This made me laugh, and I may have snorted, just a little. She got it!

The following are steps to developing your Black Belt Brain:

STEP 1:

In each of you, there is a long history of self-protection. Self-preservation is vital and is innate in all of us. It is God-given and built conveniently right into your DNA, and you don't even have to work for it. It really is the lazy man's natural black belt. The fact is that it is built in each of us to protect ourselves from harm, predators, and danger.

Developing Your Black Belt Brain

Self-preservation does not start when we are ten-months old with a sensei telling us to wax on or wax off as we fall down a flight of stairs for the first time. We just know to protect what will keep us alive. It is magical! Yes, it hurts to fall down the stairs, but when a child lands at the bottom of a flight of stairs and the tears are wiped away, we realize that they magically put their hands in the right place to protect their neck, head, heart, and lungs. This is a gift that we can use.

When a baby is startled, they put their hands out protecting their vital organs in their chest, neck, face, and brain. Their eyes widen to take in more information. This can be witnessed on Youtube. I may have spent way too much time "researching" and laughing at these videos. This self-preservation does not diminish over time, it sticks with you through adulthood and into old age. When an adult is attacked or surprised, what does that look like? Similar to a baby's reaction with no training or experience. The reactions may be slower or more deliberate, but the process is the same. We will naturally protect the vital organs that keep us living and breathing, and we will push away from the danger that is coming at us. We already have hard-wired into us a God-given power to protect ourselves.

A great example of this natural instinct happened to my son on the school playground. The phone rang from my son's school. The caller ID said the name of the school, and honestly, by now I had the phone number programmed in. I was a bit nervous before answering. I thought I was getting yet another call about running in the halls or throwing paper airplanes at inappropriate times in class. "Is this Bailey's Dad?" "Yes, what did he do now?" I found myself saying a bit too sarcastically knowing that I had a boy with my genes locked in a concrete box with windows for about eight hours a day. "Well, Mr. Mercer you see, Bailey was playing on the playground and fell. We think maybe he did something to his arm." I questioned if they had rubbed dirt in it and put a bandaid on the booboo. Then the principal said, "No, you should meet us at the doctor's office right away!" "Oh! That kind of booboo. Got it! Be right there." I felt stupid.

I quickly drove to the doctor's office that was conveniently across from the school and met with the nurse, doctor, playground attendant, and his mother, who had gotten the same call. I'm sure she handled the call better though. The doctor had just placed Bailey's arm down in his lap. Bailey lifted it up again to proudly show me what had happened and how cool it looked. He had an extra elbow where his forearm was! I had to have a seat. It looked awful!

The playground attendant told me she happened to see what had happened. Bailey was swinging from the monkey bars on the playground and fell forward, landing on his arm. She said that it looked like he was going to hit his head and that would have been horrible, but he put his arm out at the last second, which protected his head but broke the arm. I still cringe a little bit thinking about it.

I asked the doctor what would have happened if he hadn't have put his arms out. The doctor said, "You see his arm?" "Yes," I said with a grimace. "That might have been his neck," replied the doctor. Monkey bars are no joke at schools. Multiple injuries happen each year on monkey bars and playground equipment. I think they are great fun and a good demonstration here about your natural black belt speedy reactions that your body has to protect its vital organs.

This isn't a proclamation about how bad monkey bars are at school. I don't expect to see blasphemous social media posts about the terrors that monkey bars are placing on our helpless children in our school system. This is a lesson in self-protection and how you are built to protect yourself. The monkey bars are not the villain, but the arm and your natural black belt brain is a hero for protecting the brain, and the neck in this case.

That Black Belt Brain power will now become a conscious part of your training and protection experience. We already have a Black Belt Brain that is ready for action.

STEP 2:

The second step in developing your Black Belt Brain is knowing that there are two options. Option one is knowing that violence exists, and you can choose to do something about it if you are confronted. Option two is knowing that there is violence in the world and choosing to stick your head in the sand and ignore the problem or the potential problem.

I would suggest that you have already picked option one and that you are ready to prepare yourself to do something about a violent incident should it reveal itself in your personal space.

STEP 3:

Find your "why."

As police officers, we are trained to do what it takes to go home to our families and not let the bad guy win. An exercise to reinforce this is simple. Decide right now what you have to live for. Write it down, give it a name if you need to. Do this experiment with me and see if it will change your attitude and give you the size of the fight that Mark Twain was talking about.

In the academy, we were asked to make a list of what we were willing to die for: the list for me was absolutely nothing, zero, zip, zilch. Dying is unacceptable; I can do no good for my family or my family's future if I am dead.

I made a list of what I was willing to live for and what I would fight with all my might for. Here is what it looked like.

What I Live For:
- Family: Jenny, Bailey, Parker.
- I will fight with my brothers of the thin blue line so that they can go home to their families.

A short list, I know. You were probably expecting that I wanted to live for sprinkled doughnuts and maple bars with bacon strips crunched up on top. You are partially right, I do enjoy a good doughnut (I am a cop). However, I can live without those fat pills and my "why" consists only of my family.

Your list does not need to be extravagant or fancy, written in cursive or put to song lyrics, unless that is your thing. The list has to boil down to YOUR why and what you want to live for. Your list does, in fact, need to mean something special and be at the top of your mind as you go through your training and your life. It needs to give you a rock, a foundation, and a reason to survive. You absolutely can pick God, your country, property, fur babies, and your Nana if you want to. This is your list. Make it your own pride and joy but make it. Even though it may only be in your mind's eye, there is power in knowing why you need to survive. Make the list so that you know beyond a shadow of a doubt why you will keep your awareness and safety top of mind.

Your "why" is your will to survive and is your "size of the fight in the dog." Own it!

Originally, I had put in my list my department and the people I serve in my community, but I took that out because I had to take a hard, realistic look at being just a number, and a police officer is a job. After I am gone they will replace me; I am a number. That line in my statement meant nothing. Of course, I will fight the evil that reigns down on the community that I serve, but I won't step into something without knowing that I will go home to my family and neither should you. Build your list with items that matter.

STEP 4:

The fourth step in developing your Black Belt Brain is giving yourself permission to do physical damage to a real, live, breathing person. This permission does not come lightly or easily. You have to take a hard look at yourself and ask if you are worth it. Do not second guess yourself; you are worth it! God has given you life and breath and a reason to be on this planet. Own that you are worth protecting. Own that protecting yourself is worth it so that you can be there for others and the things to come in your life, in your future. You are worth it.

If you have made the decision, you have your reason and your why. You know that you and your family are worth it.

The next logical step is knowing that if an aggressor does bad things to you, he will do bad things to others. Know that this opportunity that you are given may not only be the opportunity for you to go home, but for the aggressor to stop his behavior permanently and re-think his actions for the future.

Make the violence stop with you! Take that ownership. This is not the ownership of the aggressor's problem, but the ownership to stop the problem where he stands, with you.

If you suffer from low self-worth or low self-esteem, then let me give you permission to tell yourself that you are worth it. You deserve to survive. You deserve to win. You deserve to live a life that is pain-free from the anguish that comes from beating yourself up because you didn't do what you know you should have done. You are worth it. Give yourself permission to stand up for yourself.

When a bad guy enters your space, your Trouble Bubble, and threatens you, if you do nothing, you will perpetuate the situation for others. He has just learned that he can get away with it. The anguish comes from not doing what you know you should have done to take care of the situation. That can rot at you for years in the future.

Make the decision now to give yourself permission to do damage to a live, breathing, human being if necessary and appropriate for you to survive.

Congratulations, you are starting to develop your Black Belt Brain. Good work!

Developing Your Black Belt Brain

Developing a 360 Awareness

Every police officer has to go through the basic police academy to become a full-time officer. The basic academy is just that; it gives you the basics for doing your job and for keeping yourself safe. One of the topics taught is awareness. The topic did not have a classroom or a name as such but was drilled into our heads and psyche by repetition outside of the classroom environment. It mostly happened by surprise.

One of the many tools that the academy stresses is awareness. We are not talking about some new-fangled criss-cross-applesauce, hold your hands in your lap and chant ole-bolle with a jumble of heavy vowel movements for a half a day to find your true inner-peace officer.

We are talking about the kind of awareness that can save your life and one that we all have built into us — an archaic primal awareness of trouble that has been lost because of generation iPhone. Don't get me wrong, I love my iPhone, but it will not save my life if a burglar jumps out to nab me from the dark shadows unless, however, you have the extremely rare tactical cell phone case with the app from the

App Store for $5.99 that does that very magical thing? Don't look for it. It does not exist, sorry.

With the advent of new technology such as cell phones and wearable gadgets that beep, buzz, toot, and squirt at us for everything from hitting a special walking milestone to notifying us when our neighbors are ovulating, our attention is often divided. Our attention is for sure shortened to our immediate personal proximity. We have reached a time that we could call "multi-generational-gadgetry." (I'm working on trademarking that phrase so that you will have to give me ten cents every time you use it). The gadgets of distraction exist for every generation; it is not just the young folks who are clueing out.

We are increasingly entrapped by the gadgets that are within a three to five-foot range of our bodies and are becoming extremely unbalanced about touching or paying attention to what is outside that range. Not sure you believe me? Alexa, buy me 24 of my favorite golf balls… "Ok, done Josh… they are due to arrive on the 26th, anything else?" Yes, Alexa? Can you do something about that masked home invader breaking into my back sliding glass door right now? "Ok, Josh I'll order you the new movie *Masked Home Invader*, it is due to arrive on the 26th with your other order, anything else?" No, Alexa… I'm dead, but if you could notify my lawyer and have the insurance policy paid up, my family would like my life insurance money probably by tomorrow.

Developing a 360 Awareness

"Ok, Josh. Sorry, you are dead. I'll pay everything up for you, enjoy your movie."

We used to look off into the distance to make sure that a saber tooth tiger was not lurking in the distance to make us his tasty treat before his afternoon nap under a shade tree.

Now, we may not have the saber tooth tiger lingering in the distance, but we have other critters that can jump out and entangle us without warning. There are those pesky curbs that get in the way before stepping up on the sidewalk, the water fountain that wasn't there last week, or yes, even the bad guy that wants your wallet, purse, or spare change so he can buy a beer at 8:30a.m. while you are rushing to your job.

If you have an hour, (or twelve) search on YouTube for "people walking with cell phones." This is an amazing series of videos to watch and giggle your way through those boring corporate meetings. To watch other people fail in what you and I know we have done as well, is a wonderful thing worthy of an afternoon, or at least during the long drawn out meeting you were supposed to be taking notes in.

We have all walked into something when we should have been paying attention to what was in front of us. I once walked into a screen door with a full plate of food while looking straight at it. The experience was embarrassing but awesome! I am glad there was no video of it at the time.

The experience of gawking at people on YouTube from the comfort of your easy chair walking into lakes, doors,

Developing a 360 Awareness

posts, and fountains from all over the globe is an outstanding laugh riot! This is not just a North American thing, this is happening all over the globe.

Our attention is switching swiftly over the last few years from watching where we are going to hoping we make it while we read and reply to that last-second tweet.

We seldom look out over the horizon to see where we are going and watch for the predatory cat. We would rather be paying attention to a device that is in our hands and not knowing where we are going at all but paying attention to the latest cat video with a million hits on social media.

Even though there is an app that will give us walking directions, there is not one to remind us to avoid the curb, pothole or man-hole. And there is certainly not an application that lets you know when there is a bad guy lurking around the corner ready to do you harm in exchange for a dollar, so he can afford a cold 32 oz can of Keystone Lite to get his morning drunk on.

Which brings me to the point of awareness. You can not be aware of any kind of danger lurking in the bushes or even straight ahead of you if you have your eyes bulging at your latest Instagram post or the random thumbs up, peach, air burst comment emoji on that hilarious post that you posted on social media while driving to the mall to hang with your bestie. (I know, in advance that I am not hip and am about as a saltine as they come. I do the best I can with the modern

Developing a 360 Awareness

lingo presented and limited knowledgeable use of the urban dictionary. I do have kids, I hear things).

The academy taught critical awareness by having people jump out at us from unsuspecting places and at unsuspecting times. We were not initially aware that there was anything wrong with our awareness and were happy to be just walking freely without a TAC officer yapping at us about the thread that was dangling off of the pocket of our freshly ironed shirt. Then, BANG out of nowhere was a threat from a sunken-in, shadowed door, classroom, or around a blind corner. Then there were the required pushups and butterfly kicks for not having a 360 awareness. This, of course, made us hyper-aware and anything that moved would be squashed like a bug.

I remember coming home after a grueling week at the academy and my son, Parker, jumped from behind a door to scare me as I walked through. Ironically, I had seen him through the crack and knew he was there thanks to my training. I thought he was politely opening the door for me. What good kids we have, I thought! However, I did not expect that he was going to jump out at me in an attempt to scare me. I thought he was there to help. I did jump! Which was the intended effect, but I also shot in and put him on the ground before he had time to gloat in his amazing scariness. We had to have a family conference after apologizing and dusting off the innocence of a cool 10-year-old.

Developing a 360 Awareness

Another thing the academy teaches police officers is the concept of looking around you and keeping a 360 view of your environment, not just what is out in front of you, but what is on the sides and behind you. It was for our safety, not for their entertainment that they would put us into scenarios and would challenge us to be aware of our surroundings. Everything in our surroundings we had to own.

Although I would admit that they did have a good time making sure that we had our wits about us at all times. I can't blame them, it would be fun to scare the new wide-eyed baby cops. I am still not sure if the challenge was to get us to wet ourselves or to give us special awareness powers. I believe that it was both.

Believe it or not, there are people out there who want to do officers harm because of what we do. They may not have liked getting arrested and forgot to take ownership of the bad things that they did in order to get arrested in the first place. An officer may have been human and spoke gruffly to someone, and now they hold a grudge for a lifetime. Or, an officer may have arrested their mother, brother, or girlfriend; the excuses and reasons are vast, but it comes down to a moment an officer is not paying attention to their environment so they can get revenge. We have to prepare for that instance in every situation we have.

Developing a 360 Awareness

So, how can you practice and develop awareness without going to the academy and having people appear out of nowhere to threaten you? Do you hire a scare coach?

This is probably the hardest thing to develop mentally. I suggest that you become very curious and conscious of your space and what you do with it at first.

First of all, you will need to put your cell phone in your pocket or your purse and put it on vibrate. You can check your phone after you walk because you are safe. Or, if you are super brave, try putting your cell phone on the kitchen counter and go for a walk without it. I know this is scary, but you can do it. I have faith in you.

Walk around the block and notice things around your space as you walk. Notice all the way down the block things that you have not noticed before. Keep your eye on the horizon while you notice stop signs, bushes, trees, flowers, yard signs, good people, bad people, things out of place, and things exactly where they should be. Be a noticer.

Articulate out loud the things that you notice on your walk. A side note to saying things that you notice out loud is that everyone will think YOU are the crazy one and avoid you! Do not write down what you notice anywhere and do not memorize them. The items are irrelevant; the noticing is what you will need to lock into. You want to notice things that are out on the horizon and not within your immediate stepping space. Your peripheral vision will take care of you.

Developing a 360 Awareness

You will want to hear sounds that you can identify, such as a barking dog, lawnmowers in the distance, cars coming from in front or behind you, and steps of people coming up behind you.

You will want to dart your eyes in a random triangle. Front as far as you can see. Left or right and back out to the front. You can also glance behind you and acknowledge anything that is coming up from the backside of you. If you do this real fast, you will look "special," and nobody will want to be your friend. If you do this slowly with little head movement, it will look casual and natural. The only weird thing that people will notice is that you don't have a phone in your hand. *Wow! That is unnatural; they must be aware of their surroundings, I won't pick on that person. He will see me coming from a mile away.* Yes, yes you will!

Learn to be conscious and aware of as large of a space as possible and identify everything. You could call it going into your inner "Jason Bourne Moment" where you know everything in your space. As your space and awareness grows, so will your safety.

Let's say after you do this exercise, you are walking along minding your own business, and you notice about two blocks ahead that there is a creepy, unkempt dude doing the tweaker shuffle and carrying a baseball bat. He is randomly swinging the bat in the air, and you can see that he is yelling and increasingly agitated at what you can only assume is a

Developing a 360 Awareness

mannequin in a store display window. You now can identify that you may not want to enter into this area ahead without at least a plan of attack. But more likely than not, you will not enter the area in the first place. You cross the street and continue walking and observing the trouble brewing from the opposite side of the street where there are four lanes of vehicles and space in-between you and the wacko druggie. You congratulate yourself and pat yourself on the back saying, "Whew! I just avoided being beaned in my head for the two dollars cash I have in my wallet... good job me!"

Next, you are walking alone on a bike trail, wondering why you forgot your bike, but realizing that you still need exercise to melt off that apple fritter you downed at the doughnut shop, so you decide to walk on the bike trail anyway. You notice about two miles into your walk that you have not seen anyone in a long time. You also notice that about 300 yards ahead you see a bush wiggle and a head tuck back inside the wiggly bush. You proudly turn around while getting out your cell phone to call the police to check the area. Again, you are proud that you have averted a bad situation. You buy yourself another congratulatory doughnut at Twisters Doughnut Hut on the way home... good job you! Exercise later at the gym to work off the extra carbs.

In both of the situations above you may have been fine pushing forward and walking into the potential for trouble.

But it may not have been fine, either. The bat wheedling meth junkie, commonly known as a tweaker, could have passed you by and not given you a second glance because he was busy arguing with the mannequin in the store window. Your bush buddy could have been a teenager using the bathroom at an inappropriate time or waiting to scare a buddy that was riding the trail ahead of you. Regardless of the outcome, you will be safer noticing and having the choice of avoiding the potential of danger rather than being completely unaware of it in the first place and having it catch you off guard. We don't like surprises.

The other place that you can practice is the common places you travel or shop. If you go into a grocery store with your head in your phone or in the shopping list that you have created so that you won't have to come back yet again to pick up that one or two items, you may be missing a huge opportunity to work on your 360 awareness. Look around you and notice all the people with green shirts. You can even make a game of it with your kids if you have young children. Just be careful to give what you are finding a name like "green shirt" rather than blurting out "THERE'S ONE!" Because it is inevitable that someone will not appreciate being pointed out and they will think that you are pointing at their enlarged muffin top or the color of their skin or the freakishly large feet they have a complex about.

Developing a 360 Awareness

The supermarket drill may make your shopping trip a little longer, but safety isn't just convenient; it could save your life. You are still developing your black belt mind and awareness. By increasing your awareness space that is outside of your three to five-foot area, you will also be able to avoid crashing supermarket carts and bumping into people, unless you are into that kind of thing.

You can add in or complicate the grocery store exercise by tuning into the elevator music and naming the tune that is playing on the overhead speakers. You will also earn bonus points by listening for a shopping cart that has a wobbler for a wheel, but that is an advanced safety move. I will be the one pushing the cart. I inevitably get that cart. I always forget that I can test drive them before I load up.

The practicality of the above exercise is to expand the awareness of your surroundings, which may not only help you from bumping into people but may also save your life in the future because you are no longer just aware of your three to five foot personal bubble.

Let's say that after you develop your 360 awareness for a couple of months that you are walking from a theater to your car. You say goodbye to your friends and part ways. Your friends found rock star parking right next to the theater doors. They are rude and took off right after you said goodbye. They have reviews to post about the buttered popcorn, and Diet Coke served at the movie, it cannot wait any longer, and their cell phone is at a critical 10% go-go juice. Gotta go, Bye!

The movie was one of the last ones that evening, and the parking lot is empty except for a few spattered cars in the lot. About halfway to your car, you notice a bright amber glow in one of the cars ahead of you about 100 yards. You note that the car is uncomfortably and unusually close to your car. Your senses are heightened, you can smell the odor of cigarette smoke, and you notice several butts on the ground outside the vehicle. Why were they there so long? They must be waiting for something.

You begin to get a sense that the car has been waiting for a while. You get an uneasy feeling as you look harder into the car. You can see that there are two males and they look anxious. There is a soft glow of the overhead parking lot lights that light up the inside of the car just enough to see that they are looking at you as you close the gap. Even though you have pepper spray and a knife in your purse, you don't chance it. You turn around and head back to the theater where you hope to find a burly security guard that can walk you to your car. As you turn around to head back to the theater, you hear the click of two car doors. You nonchalantly glance over your shoulder and notice that one of the males is holding something in his hand like rope or twine. You make a run for the movie theater and to safety. Congratulations, you have avoided being attacked.

Developing a 360 Awareness

The simple fact of being aware outside your own three to five feet of comfort zone will keep you safer than if you don't put awareness into your routine.

Practice being aware of your surroundings and do not be afraid to trust your intuition. Your intuition is there to do a job. Its job is to keep you safe and give you early warning signs. If your gut tells you that something is wrong, something is wrong. If your gut and intuitions are wrong, then you are still right for trusting it.

There is no harm done in turning around on a trail or crossing the street to a safer location or even going back into your office building to have someone walk out to your car with you because you have an uneasy feeling. There is a reason for it. The hair stands up on the back of your neck for a reason. The reason is right. Trust it.

There is no shame in avoiding trouble to avoid violence, but you cannot do it if you are not aware of your surroundings. Keep your head on a swivel and keep aware of your space. Become your own Jason Bourne and begin to Think like a Cop.

Developing a 360 Awareness

Body Language

Your body tells a story in language that is not verbal. Body language is simply a physical, behavioral action that corresponds with your mood, attitude, being, and internal thoughts and feelings, as opposed to the words that we use to express our everyday concepts and information. Body language is communication without the use of those pesky guttural noises that escape our mouths before offending someone.

Body language is what you wish your three-year-old would use more of when she sees a scary snake or unknown critter in the house instead of breaking your wine glass with the high pitched squeal. You think out loud, "Perhaps we can enroll her in singing lessons, and she can pay our mortgage in a few years" as you comment to your wife who is pulling her finger out of her bloody ear.

Body language includes facial expressions, eye movement, body postures, and positioning. Gestures both large and minuscule communicate our intentions, mood, and what we are trying to say with our verbal language, it is just manifested in our bodies in the form of expression. We

Body Language

don't realize how much we communicate with our bodies. Facial expressions and general movement are automatic and ingrained in our patterns until we are made consciously aware of how we are using this obscure form of communication.

If you are nervous, you will show it on your person. Think in your mind's eye for a moment of someone who is nervous when they talk in front of a group of people. I would suggest putting the person on a large screen T.V. in your mind. On one half of the T.V is the person with bad posture and nervous ticks. Imagine the posture that they must have to communicate unconsciously to articulate their nervousness.

Now, think of someone who is confident and proficient at being in front of a group of people. Put this person on the other side of the T.V screen. In your mind's eye, you can see their posture and body language. The body language of someone who is confident is someone we will gravitate to.

Because you are running an imagination station in your head and broadcasting your image to the T.V., imagine those two people communicating a story, the same story, and without sound; all they can do is talk with their bodies. They are telling a story of the largest fish they ever caught. Who do you want to believe? Who do you want to interrupt? Who do you want to tell to get to the point or you may even hear someone say, "Prove it... do you have a picture?" Both videos are playing in vivid color, yet one side is awkward and cumbersome, you want them to be confident or just leave the situation. The other video you will be more drawn to and want to pay attention to what they have to say. They are both communicating the same story about the largest fish they ever caught, but you are drawn to one, you believe one, and you may even question the other because his body language is incongruent with his story.

We cannot help but leak our feelings into our communication whether we want it to or not. It happens on a subconscious level until you are conscious of it. You can then change your body language to tell another more purposeful and powerful story. People, in fact, want you to be more confident, they are waiting for it. People will naturally gravitate toward confidence. This is not a confidence course. However, we need to understand how not to be a target, which is where confidence comes into play.

In our example above with the confident speaker and the nervous speaker, who would be more likely to be challenged? The nervous speaker in a conversation, right? The same thing is true for when you are walking down the street or standing with your shopping bags loading your car. The person who is walking and communicating that they are shy and nervous will get picked out by a predictor because the predator believes they can take them. If they are not aware of their surroundings, they may even be able to take them by surprise, which will give an attacker an extra edge. Why? Because they lack the confidence to protect themselves for one. They may not even have the confidence to yell out for help. A criminal will pick the least likely person to cause him or her difficulties. I do not want this to be you if it can be helped with a little body language switch-a-roo.

Our physical expression can tell a lot about what we are trying to communicate. The current leading theory was developed by a cool cat in the 1960s and 70s by the name of Albert Mehrabian. I picture him with a plaid scarf, a light brown coat with dark brown patches on the elbows, a pipe smelling of cherry tobacco, and ironically, talking a lot with his hands and facial expressions. The theory is that 55% of communication is body language, 38% is the tone of voice, and 7% is actually the spoken word. If that is the case, then over half of our communication is body language and yet we spend little time learning about it.

I spent my formative, growing up years in Canada and English was my second language. I used that line a lot when I moved back to America because spelling on some things are different, such as colour instead of color. My English teacher in America was understanding, but evidently, I still needed to understand what those universal pesky nouns and verbs were and where to put them in a sentence. I used that joke in an interview for a police department when they asked

Body Language

if I spoke a second language. I told them I spent several years in Canada and I speak the language fluently. I didn't get the job; it was a joke they didn't fully appreciate. Maybe I should have mimed it? Maybe I should have added the punch line that I also speak body language?

Because body language is such an important part of our communication with each other, I have spent some extended time analyzing what works with police officers when communicating with bad guys and what does not.

I began looking at officers that were fresh out of the academy. I looked at them and noticed that they did not look as confident and solid as the officers who had been on the police force for an extended time. I noticed that they stood differently, held their hands differently, and their posture was different. But what was different? I took a mental picture of three different types of officers and analyzed the differences. This picture seemed to be universal across several departments and agencies.

The first type of officer was a seasoned officer; he had a wide stance that was different than the average citizen. He stood with his chest forward, shoulders back. His back was straight, knees slightly bent, and he balanced on the balls of his feet. The toes of his feet were slightly articulated to the outside of his body. His stance was slightly wider by an inch or two than his shoulders.

He maintained this solid stance even when he wasn't talking with a suspect or a citizen. This made his stance natural at all times; he looked comfortable. When he was talking with a citizen, they listened intently to what he had to say. The ironic thing was that he may not even be well spoken. However, he had a stage presence that was tangible. When he spoke, everyone stopped to listen because it was going to be important, even if it wasn't.

When the seasoned officer talked and even when he didn't, he had his hands outstretched at about chest level and he was doing something with them, like taking notes or had his hands in a type of praying motion as he touched the tips of his fingers together. He would play with his fingers and thumbs to give himself something to do, but his hands were always there, up in a calm and steady area in front of his chest. As he talked, he gently gestured. He didn't fidget with his hands and fingers, he just moved them in slow motion as he spoke. The slower the motion, the calmer he seemed.

The second type of officer had about a year or two working as a police officer. This type of officer had made it out of the academy and off of the field training phase. This meant that he was able to be in his own car and did not have to be babysat through his calls. He was his own man and out doing police work by himself.

This second type of police officer had an upright stance, his feet were about shoulder width apart, and he stood flat-footed or slightly on the balls of his feet. He stood with his hands resting on his hips or up by his chest. He would balance back and forth on one hip or the other, like a gentle, slow, uncomfortable dance in middle school only all by himself. When you think about it, most of middle school was a dance of partial awkwardness sprinkled in with bits of awesome, just as this juvenile officer is practicing. He is trying to find what works for him in his stance and readiness. He is well-spoken and articulate, however when he spoke with bad guys or citizens, they may or may not have paid attention to him and what he had to say based on his trial and error stance and body positioning.

The second officer type didn't look uncomfortable but looked like he was trying to find a balance.

The third type of police officer was fresh out of the academy and stood with a narrow stance, shallower than the other two, with one of his legs bent slightly, and he stood on his heels, not on the balls of his feet. It also seemed that this type of officer was arched forward or slumped at the upper back ever so slightly as if he was listening really hard. He stood with his hands in or just outside of his pockets below the waist or just at the belt line, maybe with his thumbs tucked into his belt. This officer may cross his arms at his chest but would not seem to talk with his hands much at this level. His feet were rigid and at about an inch under shoulder width apart. This third type of officer may lock one leg straight and angle the other. He is very casual and unassuming, however, looked almost nervous or intimidated as he would talk with a suspect.

The third type of police officer had an average citizens' stance; very unassuming. He usually angled one foot to one side or the other, and the other foot he pointed straight. His hands were mostly down to his sides, and when he did talk with his hands, the gestures were shallow, and it looked like he was embarrassed to use them. His hands barely made it up to chest level when he spoke; it seemed to leave him open and unprotected when compared to the other two types of officers. He was well-spoken and articulate, but soft-spoken in confidence.

When the third type of officer spoke with bad guys, they would pick him apart. This type of officer was often called names by the guys he was trying to arrest. It was not uncommon for a criminal to call this type of officer a rookie and question his authority. Even though he may technically say the right thing, a career criminal would eat him alive in a verbal joust. This type of officer would need a seasoned officer to step in and take over a conversation. The seasoned officer would step in and take over knowing that with time the new officer would learn how to communicate better, just as he had learned over time.

Upon noticing these differences, I began to play with them to make sense of what I saw in the petri dish of clientele

Body Language

I had to work with. At first, I stood like the third officer: narrow, hunched, and on my heels. The female I was dealing with would not give me her name and kept playing games with me until finally she bolted and a short foot chase ensued. That experiment ended badly, but I pressed on to find body language answers.

Next, after some failed attempts at playing officer number three, I tried the same approach and then about mid conversation switched to officer number one in my stance and hand placement. I immediately got great feedback. Historical liars and villains began stopping in their tracks and paying attention. I had no more foot pursuits. No more long, drawn-out conversations to get the required information and fewer people would argue and fight. My assertion was that it was simple body language and congruent facial expressions, the 55% that I was not saying to the person in front of me, that made all the difference.

When our facial expressions and body language are congruent and are talking the same language that is coming out of our mouths, we will make more sense to the people we are talking with. I actually had fewer fights when I stood differently and held my hands differently than the general population. What kind of sorcery was this? This was magical. I had to share it.

I contacted a new recruit and told him about my amazing discovery. I believe I framed it something like, "You have to try this non-verbal hocus-pocus magic mumbo-jumbo that I just discovered." (Because I'm pretty technical that way). Once he tried it, he became a convert. The strange thing about it was that others in the department started to view him as an experienced officer as well. I noticed that out of the blue citizens and criminals would turn to him for the answers that they would normally have and naturally turned to a seasoned officer for. I believed that I had broken the code. I just about broke my arm patting myself on the back thinking that I invented something special. I didn't; it has always been there.

How can you emulate a state of power and authority like a seasoned officer in a time of uncertainty? Maybe there is the threat of violence, and you want to dissipate it quickly? You may just want to project more authority in your everyday life when you walk to your car. You can project yourself with authority and awareness that we have already discovered so that you don't get picked out and targeted.

You may even want people to listen more intently or to pay attention to you in a board meeting. If this is the case, try doing the following until you get the results you are looking for.

BODY LANGUAGE BASICS

STEP 1:

Widen feet to about an inch or two outside of your shoulders, balance on the balls of your feet, and bend your knees slightly to give the appearance that you are well-balanced and have a solid foundation yet are ready to spring into action. This is subtle; you do not want to be running around on your tippy toes, just slightly balanced on the ball of your feet.

You will also want to do what is called "blading your stance," meaning that you want to have one foot slightly forward by about three to five inches, depending on how tall you are. This stance, when you look in the mirror, because I know you will be doing that, will appear athletic, naturally balanced, calm yet confident, and casually ready for action.

Now that you have the stance down you can test it by narrowing your stance and having your significant other push your shoulder from the front. You may easily lose balance backward with your old stance.

Widen your feet again and blade your stance. This may feel a bit awkward at first, but when your pushing partner gives you a little push from the front, you will feel more grounded and solid in your presence.

Body Language

STEP 2:

Stand straight, look straight at the problem or issue, puff out your chest slightly but don't look like you are puffing out your chest. Hold yourself tall. Stand with your back straight, not hunched forward like you are leaning into the wind. Your back should be directly above your torso. Your shoulders should be back and relaxed. Lean slightly forward and look like you are ready for a child to walk up and give you a gentle nudge in the middle of your chest.

Hmmm, didn't phase me tiny child, neiner neiner!

STEP 3:

Talk naturally with your hands and arms out in front of your chest. Talk calmly with your hands, don't just flail around like an inflatable happy flappy sky dancing man used for cheesy advertising on a busy street to garner the attention of passers-by. Have some poise and dignity, man!

Speak calmly with your hands at about chest high and your elbows relaxed at your sides. Your gestures do not need to be outrageous unless you are talking about that fish you hauled in yesterday and you want to distract from the fact that it was actually a minnow.

Pick a few hand and arm gestures that will seem natural to your audience while you speak. Find a resting gesture that still keeps your hands in front of your chest even though you are not currently speaking.

The three resting phases I see used most often are: Folding of their hands palm to palm then switch to touching the tips of the fingers together in an arrow or spear formation toward the person experienced officers are talking with, then loosely interlace the bottom three fingers with both hands clasped together. (The two pointer fingers will still be pointed as a spear toward their audience, and their two thumbs will be touching the tips.) It almost looks like a loose James Bond pose with their fingers pointed forward instead of up at the sky. They typically articulate their fingers toward the people or audience they are speaking with.

Ok, I can hear you say, *how will all of this finger-pointing and gesturing with praying hands by my chest keep me safe?*

Glad you asked!

We are born with the innate ability to protect ourselves when something bad happens. When something bad does happen, and someone takes a swing at you out of the blue, what area are your hands in?

YES! Exactly Right!

Your arms and hands will be in the perfect spot to defend your vital organs in your chest and head. Your arms will be in place to keep the bad guy from hitting your head and knocking you out. Your arms and hands will be in the perfect place for protecting your heart and lungs from damage which will, in turn, give you time to react and stay in the fight. Keep in mind that if you get knocked out, the game is over and the bad guy can have his way with you.

Your hands and arms will be in the perfect area for a quick block or quick defense. Your hands will know instinctively what to do and what area to cover for defense, just as if you were ten months old and fell down the stairs. Once you have mounted your instinctive self-defense, you can launch an offense to get out of the situation. You cannot do that if you are on the pavement in a puddle.

If you had your hands in your nice comfy jean pockets or looped all cool-like in your belt loops like you are posing for senior pictures in the 1980s or stuck in your pockets because you want to appear all casual and chill, it will take your body's natural black belt reaction time longer to get your hands and arms into a place of protection. It may be too late. Microseconds count.

Spend some time practicing the above steps in the privacy of your own home in front of a full-length mirror. If you don't have a full-length mirror, go buy one and invest in some self-preservation. You will feel awkward at first but keep at it. Take bits and pieces to work with you to practice at the water cooler during casual conversations to find out what works for you and what doesn't.

Practice before you need to have the look of a seasoned police officer in a potentially violent situation. In fact, the reason a seasoned police officer looks seasoned is that he has spent many years perfecting his craft. He did not have a book to tell him how to short circuit the system. You have to become invested with time, practice, and experimentation to find what will work for you and fit in your life.

What I can tell you for certain is that if your body language and your verbal content stay congruent when you tell someone to get back, or there is going to be hell to pay, they will believe you and back off.

Go practice and make it perfect for you.

Body Language

Verbal Jiu-Jitsu and De-Escalation

I was watching interviews a few years ago with what I believe was a high-level Jiu-Jitsu practitioner and fighter. He said that people want to fight him all the time because he is a famous fighter and one of the founding fathers of American Jiu-Jitsu. I imagine that people want to test his skills all the time. He said something to the effect of, "People don't mind losing to someone they know can hurt them really bad because they will get some sort of strange fame from it. An ego boost, if you will. Also, if they do get hurt and lose, they would now have something to brag about for the rest of their lives."

I would imagine a story like, "Yeah, I have this permanent limp because I lost a fight to this amazing guy, it was incredible!" The story would go on, "I could have beat him, but the sun was in my eyes." It was a win-win for the fools who would want to take the fighter on, and a lose-lose for the seasoned fighter and brand name he was attempting to build at the time.

The fighter was, and is, a genius and a beast on the mat. He would never turn down an opportunity to fight in a dojo or in the street if it was a real threat. This man hurts people for a living, and he trains others to hurt people. He has built a brand and a name for modern martial arts in America and the world with Jiu-Jitsu. However, he was not willing to trade that for an inconsequential chest bumping match with a drunk at a bar. In fact, I believe he told the interviewer that he would not put himself in that situation in the first place. But, he did continue with the interview.

What the fighter said next in the interview struck me as probably the smartest thing a fighter has ever said in regard to the de-escalation of a fight.

The fighter was asked by the interviewer for his advice about a bar scene and was given a scenario about being approached by someone who was intoxicated and wanted to fight. He was asked something to the effect of, "What is the one self-defense move you would use if someone approached you in a bar and demanded to fight?"

He confidently said the best line I have ever heard come out of a fighter's mouth ever; he said, "You win!" As simple as this sounds it is also very complex. As he said, "You win!" he put both his hands up a little higher than chest level and his palms were toward the threat. He articulated his forearms out at about a 45-degree angle and splayed his fingers open. He said it with a smile on his face that was genuinely friendly, not smug or sarcastic. I thought the interview was amazing and his answer to the question was

Verbal Jiu-Jitsu and De-Escalation

brilliant and simple. There are some body science and verbal suggestions that are in place that are worth some exploration.

This was several years ago that I watched this, so I hope I do the explanation justice. I attempted to find the interview on YouTube because everything is on there. It was gone. Even all of Google didn't have a clue where this interview went. The following are the highlights as best as I can remember:

The reason for the answer the fighter gave for using the language he did was that it gave the person threatening to fight him an ego boost. They just won a battle with a prizefighter that hurts people for money in the ring. How amazing is it that he didn't get his skull crushed? They believe that they had defeated someone without really trying, they must be really powerful and special. The fighter gave the testosterone junkie something to feed on.

While the drunken fool was munching on a side of think-about-it sauce, the fighter was protecting himself with his hands and arms. He raised his hands about shoulder height and staggered them toward the intoxicated fight-requester making the threat.

The interviewer with the questions was now playing the bad guy in an impromptu bad acting clinic. The interviewer couldn't help but smile a little because he got it right away. It did feel good to win against a legend in the ring. The

Verbal Jiu-Jitsu and De-Escalation

interviewer knew that he would not have a chance otherwise. He was grateful for the gift of winning without trying.

The second reason was the MMA fighter brought his hands up just above the chest, high and prepared to fight in a non-threatening way. But he did this without clenching his fists and looking like he was going to fight. In fact, he splayed his fingers open which is extremely counter-intuitive for a fighter. He did not puff out his chest or open his arms wide in a "whatcha gonna do buddy?" motion, he closed his arms inward and kept his elbows in towards his torso. He was natural and calm, confident with a side of safe. His palms were out in a friendly manner, almost as if he was ready to receive a double high five, yet he was ready for immediate action from an attacker if there was no talking down a fool from doing this foolish errand. His hands and elbows were close to his body and provided perfect protection for his vital organs. His open fingers provided a wider coverage area that the challenger would have to navigate through.

The third was the fighter's non-verbal clues and body language that he was pushing out to the person, (interviewer in this case) asking to fight him. He is clearly athletic; he demonstrated a wide and ready stance and a hard target. The best part of the whole thing was his confident smile and non-confrontational front. The idea that the tough guy approaching him was someone who he didn't want to fight

Verbal Jiu-Jitsu and De-Escalation

(not that he couldn't take him, but that he really didn't want the spectacle up on YouTube for the world to see). So he was telling the truth by saying "You win, (I don't want to fight you)" only for different reasons than the knuckle dragger was imagining.

The Jiu-Jitsu master got to walk off unscathed in the media. Win. The foolish fighter got to keep his limbs and pride intact and gain a little fake victory. Win. No punches were thrown. Nobody got hurt. Everyone walked away a winner.

The previous chapter got into powerful body language and how to use it. The above example is how a powerful man uses body language and psychology to de-escalate a potential fight situation and walk away with a win-win and nobody even getting their feelings hurt. In fact, everybody was happy. I would imagine that the aggressor then would slap him on the back and say something to the effect of "Just kidding, lemme buy you a beer."

Now the story goes, "Hey you know that MMA guy? Well, I saw him in a bar last week, month, year, and we shared a beer together. We are besties now... great guy!" Rather than, "Dude, check out my new breathing tube!"

So how does a police officer quickly de-escalate a situation so that it doesn't end up in a fight or a potentially deadly situation?

Verbal Jiu-Jitsu and De-Escalation

The above question is up for debate because most states do not mandate a formal de-escalation type of training, yet. However, I can tell you that experienced officers will want to calm a situation quickly to get to a swift and painless resolve as soon as possible. The longer they wait, the more chances there are for a violent person to spiral out of control and hurt something or someone.

First, you will want to be mindful of verbal and body language that would suggest that the situation is going to get out of hand. If someone is telling you that they will hurt you, that is a pretty good indication that someone will follow through with those plans. Some of the non-verbal or body language gets a little tricky but after you know what you are looking for, things get a lot simpler. It is like the aggravated person is screaming things at you with his body language. Once you know the non-verbal clues, you will be able to pick them up fast when they are unfolding in front of you.

Body language that you will need to watch out for and keep a close eye on is the clenching and unclenching of someone's fists. Typically, they will do this in conjunction with dropping their hands to the sides of themselves as they try to talk themselves into violence. Of course, if you see clenched fists coming up to the front of their body and into a boxer's pose, this is obvious. However, we are talking about the subtle art of de-escalation. When someone is clenching and unclenching their fists at their sides, you

Verbal Jiu-Jitsu and De-Escalation

should be very careful because they are deciding if they want to hit you or not. It is time to back off a touch and start talking with your hands out in front of your chest.

The second thing you will want to watch for is a tightening of the jaw and tightening of the lips. A person may start pacing in feigned disgust at the situation or throw their arms around with clenched fists, tight lips, and clamped down jaw directed toward you. They are giving you an insight into their soul that says, *I am getting ready to punch you.* They are waiting for a good opportunity to get a swing in.

They are doing two things. One, they are trying to tell you that they are going to do it, and two, they are looking for you to talk them out of it or give them an outlet to leave because they don't want to fight. They are not there yet. If you trap them or if they feel trapped with no other option, they will resort to violence.

This being said, people with violent histories or people who like violence will be better at hiding these signs. Just as you will be better at looking like a police officer with your stance, posture, and what you do with your hands, they have practiced not looking like they will strike you. You will know only when their fist starts flying and you are in the way.

The third thing is The Thousand Yard Stare. As you are speaking with someone and they begin to show signs of aggression with their body language, facial expressions, and other hints that they are throwing out at you unconsciously,

Verbal Jiu-Jitsu and De-Escalation

you may also notice that the person is looking at you, but not quite at you. You may identify it as staring off into the distance a thousand yards away, right through you, even though you are looking him in the eyes.

If you are faced with an opportunity to talk with one of these people who are in an extremely heightened state, beware. The best way to deal with it, of course, is not to be there. If you can excuse yourself and leave or get out of the situation, then you should do that. If leaving is not an option, then you have to de-escalate the potentially violent person so that you can either do your job or de-escalate them enough to find an escape route for yourself. The following steps should be considered.

Keep in mind that this is a fluid encounter and you should leave or wrap things up as soon as possible. If the lines of communication are open, then keep them open. This is not about random violence but about a situation that can escalate to violence if not de-escalated.

Calm yourself before attempting to calm someone else down. If you let yourself get riled up and belligerent along with the person you are dealing with that is riled up and belligerent, then now we have two or more people who are out of control, and that will lead to a certain confrontation and physical altercation.

Take a deep breath and understand that the person in this state is out of control and you need to keep an eye on

Verbal Jiu-Jitsu and De-Escalation

him. You will want to understand that if you buy into his/her attitude, you will trigger your natural flight, fight, or freeze response, which will do things to your body that you do not want, such as shallow your breathing, pick up your heart rate, and shrink your pupils so that you can easily get tunnel vision. You want to be able to see wide and deep with normal vision so that you can judge the situation for what it is. If you trigger your freeze response, then you will be at the whim of the bad guy, and he will win because you are frozen.

Keep yourself in check with a couple of deep breaths and the realization you need to deal with this situation and be safe.

Maintain a neutral facial expression. To go with your neutral face expression, speak in a dull or calm manner. That does not mean that you should not talk with emphasis, it just means that you should talk calmer than your opposing party. You should also begin to speak in a lower, quieter level than they are so that they may have to pause and pay attention to hear you. This may break their pattern of potential violence.

Find a mutual connection. Start with attempting to find out the person's name. By finding out their name, you start to build rapport with the person quickly. Calling them by their name will enable you to begin to establish a bond with them. People naturally have a strong connection with their name. Friends and loved ones call people by their first name all the time. The quicker you can identify and call someone

Verbal Jiu-Jitsu and De-Escalation

by their first name, the quicker it will be to calm them down. Also, because you have established a possible friend, being on a first name basis, it is a lot harder to hurt someone who you are friends with than a stranger. So, become friends with them. You don't have to like them; you do have to like quickly establishing a rapport with them to de-escalate them. If things work out, you can always friend request them later on social media.

Keep in mind that you want to present a congruent front. If you become genuinely interested in their problem, they will feel it and respond easier than if the interest is fake. Find that connection. Use any common connection that you can find to talk with them about something other than what they are upset with at the time. It may be fishing, golf, hiking, the love of chocolate. Find something that is personal to the outraged savage before you. You can always come back to the reason they are upset later. This is a quick rapport trick that will help you establish a bond that could get you out of a bad situation.

Validate the person's thoughts and feelings. That does not mean that you agree with the person. Validation means that you have heard what they are trying to communicate. You can do this by paraphrasing back to them their thoughts and asking any qualifying questions to clarify how THEY are feeling about it.

Verbal Jiu-Jitsu and De-Escalation

This is an actual conversation taken from the archives of police work:

A caller stated that he could hear hissing and scratching outside his house in a nice neighborhood. He thought that a wild animal was injured and flopping up against his house. He requested police services to investigate. He said that he could hear wild thumping and hissing and crashing against his house. He was concerned about the animal but was too old to investigate himself as he was wheelchair-bound.

Upon arriving, officer Mantle found a male crouched up against the building and meowing while clawing at the siding of the house. He could immediately see what the problem was. A drug-induced personal party. As fun as this party was, it was beginning to wake up the neighborhood. When he drove up and pointed his spotlight on the male, he arched his back and hissed wildly. He then turned to hiss at the sprinkler system that kept hitting him while he went about de-clawing himself on the side of the building and the tree. While Mantle drove up, he could see neighbor's lights begin to come on in the windows surrounding the house with the troubled cat. He was clawing a tree in the yard of the nice caller's house. The male would focus on the tree or house, then get hit with the sprinkler again. He would jump and smack the house. He then attempted to climb up the tree, but alas, he was not a cat and would lose traction and fall, causing more hissing and frustration from the male (uh, cat).

Officer Mantle happen to like weird. Frankly, the weirder, the better. People are awesome, and he loved figuring out what makes them tick. He launched into a conversation with the cat. The cat (uh, human) was very scared; he was very intent on climbing the tree to get away from the pesky sprinkler that kept attacking him.

The conversation went something like this:

"I understand that you think you are a cat. You will have to agree that this is a little out of the ordinary, right?" The cat looked at the officer and hissed while wiping the hair from his forehead with his paw.

The cat shrugged and began to stand and look as though he was going to run away. At this point, the officer recognized him as one of the county regulars and ran his name through the dispatch system. He showed signs that he understood what the officer was doing by pausing and shrugging his shoulders, he also took up what the officer imagined was a cat-like fighting stance and prepared to fight (like a cat). The cat/human thought he had a warrant and was prepared to fight and scratch his way from going to jail that night. Perhaps he had mice to chase.

Officer Mantle spoke to him using his first name and advised him that he didn't have a warrant and that he could leave because he was actually trespassing on this man's property.

Verbal Jiu-Jitsu and De-Escalation

Officer Mantle also advised him that the county had a neuter law for male stray cats and didn't want him to have to go through that, as he believed that he was a man, not a cat. But the officer didn't make the rules and if the male wanted to identify as a cat… then rules are rules. With that, the cat person stood up straight and asked if he was free to go in a deep human voice. Mantle told him that he was free to go but that he needed to stay out of people's yards.

And with that, he walked off on two legs and joined the real world of humans.

By listening to this strange aberration and acknowledging that officer Mantle had heard he was a cat, he did not have to prove his point to him. He may have had a fight on his hands with a 200-pound cat (uh, human). Officer Mantle helped find a solution and an out for a trapped animal that was both good for the neighborhood and for the cat (uh, human).

Give them options or help them find options. This could be a choice of options you pick or options that they pick. Such as you can fight me, but I promise that you will be up against a hard target, or you can walk away.

As the calm person in the situation, you will have a clear vision of what your options are and what theirs are. It is up to you to communicate and give them rational options. They may only have a clear, concise, one-track mind into what they want or need to accomplish. (I want to rob, rape, kidnap,

Verbal Jiu-Jitsu and De-Escalation

and murder you). You can have a rational option like none of the above, but unless you can give them other options that include theirs, they may not hear you as being rational in their minds.

Such as: "You say you want to hurt me, John, I hear you, and that is an option, however, I'm going to fight like hell, and you will probably end up in the hospital before going to jail. I wouldn't want that for you. How about you just take off and we will call it a night." This is similar to "You win." They may actually see it as a win that they get to leave a situation.

Allow for the choice they are going to pick. You will want to pick the option for them because it will allow you not to get hurt. However, if you pick the option, then they will not own it.

"Whatever you chose is up to you John, I'm not going to pick for you. The option is up to you as to what you pick. The choice is yours. I just want you to be aware that I have options as well and I will not go easy into the night. You have the option to walk right now. The other option will hurt really bad, and you will probably have a hospital bill afterword. I don't want that for you, but if that is what you choose, then the choice is yours."

When you can say all of this with congruent body language and conviction, you have done all that you can to convince the person. Now is the time to let them decide.

Verbal Jiu-Jitsu and De-Escalation

Once they pick, they have made their choice and will reap the consequences.

Now that they have options, do not block their way of escape. Make it easy for them to walk or run away.

Verbal Jiu-Jitsu and De-Escalation

Discovering Your Trouble Bubble

Space and distance will keep you alive in a violent situation and give you a chance at survival. The more space you have, the more you will be thankful for it because the easier it will be to get away from a potential violent predator.

Your newfound awareness will help give you a profound advantage in creating and being aware of danger at a distance because you are now aware of the potential of trouble. You are also ahead of the average citizen put in the same situation.

You may want to experiment with distances to find your own personal comfort zone. I call this zone the Trouble Bubble, and it is your own personal awareness zone that you can take with you anywhere. I will give you some history of the Trouble Bubble and where its roots came from. Police officers work with safety zones on the job all the time, it keeps us safe and alive.

The Tueller Drill or The Tueller Rule is a training exercise that we used in the academy and on training days. It is used to define and forecast distance and danger. The Tueller Drill is more commonly called the twenty-one-foot rule. The twenty-one-foot rule is like it sounds. You have twenty-one feet in which to react with lethal accuracy to a subject who is bringing violence your way with a knife. The Tueller Rule used a knife as an example, but this could include anything. When facing a person with a knife, a bad guy can cover twenty-one feet and effectively do lethal damage to a police officer by cutting them in the same amount of time the police officer is able to draw and appropriately fire his weapon at the charging target.

The catch to the Tueller Rule is that the attacker has momentum and adrenaline that he has built up. Regardless of a hole in his chest, he can still inflict a major amount of pain and damage on a police officer after covering twenty-one feet. It is sad to say that many police officers have fallen to a knife or other objects meant to inflict bodily harm. It is not just damaging, it can also mean death.

In 1983, Sergeant Dennis Tueller of the Salt Lake City Utah Police Department had his findings published in SWAT magazine. The title of the article was "How Close Is Too Close?" Tueller, in his research, was curious about how fast someone could close the distance and launch a knife attack on a police officer. Tueller concluded that it would take the average male about 1.5 seconds to cover the distance of twenty-one feet. (This is without adrenaline, anger, or athleticism; this is just average time for the average person). It just so happens that 1.5 seconds is about the average time it takes a practiced police professional to draw their open, carried, holstered weapon and accurately place a bullet on a still and stationary paper target. The stationary target does not have any kind of anger, hostility, or cutting ability; the situation is rather calm.

The paper target at twenty-one feet was not a moving target who is foaming at the mouth and articulating bad thoughts in the police officer's direction. This is also not a target that has superhuman strength and pain tolerance because of the use of PCP, methamphetamine, alcohol, or an experimental dosage combination of all three with a sprinkle of natural cinnamon to make things organic. This target is just a paper shape at the end of a tape measure and a timer to ensure accuracy.

The twenty-one-foot rule was born in the 1980s but lives in police culture today. The twenty-one-foot rule is taught at every police academy and haunts most police officers as they do their jobs on the street. I would imagine that every officer on the street could articulate and pace off twenty-one feet while telling stories of its virtue. It is ingrained in police culture, yet unheard of in the ranks of citizens roaming the streets.

When I first began giving seminars on self-protection and awareness, I was in awe at how many people had not heard of this simple twenty-one-foot rule. All of the martial arts I had taken in multiple cities in America and Canada had not mentioned it. So, in retrospect, I guess I am not totally

Discovering Your Trouble Bubble

and completely surprised that I had not heard of it before entering the police academy. I have been thankful for the discovery and the time it took to get it embedded into our culture. Thank you, Mr. Tueller, good work.

I have found in my training and experience that the twenty-one-foot rule is an accurate distance for bracing yourself for violence as well. It is true when there is no knife in the equation. Distance is distance. The knife does not make the distance shrink or expand when you have a thug barreling toward you; the weapon does not seem to matter. The time it takes to brace yourself for impact or make a decision as to what you are going to do with a situation is also in play without the knife. You have one and a half seconds.

One point five seconds is very little time to mount a counter attack if someone is charging at you, even if they don't have a knife as in Tueller's example. And once they reach you, then what? If you are a citizen on the street with no weapon to defend yourself other than your wits and your hands, arms, and feet, what do you do then? Cover and turtle? Brace for impact? Fight back? Or launch a full force violence on the subject so that you can protect yourself or your family?

The choice is yours. I hope you fight for your life.

Mythbusters covered this Tueller type of drill in a 2012 episode called "Duel Dilemmas." It was proven by the

Discovering Your Trouble Bubble

Mythbusters team that at twenty feet the person with a gun was, in fact, able to get shots off at a charging attacker. The shots happened right at the time that the attacker reached the Mythbusters test subject. What the Mythbusters did not cover was that the bad guy still had momentum. With enough testosterone and pain-defying drugs in their system, the shots on a meth-induced target would take a while to take effect, and they would still be able to do a lot of damage.

If the bad guy gets in a slice with a knife on their police officer target, the police officer could be in real trouble as he is attempting to subdue the attacker. The Mythbusters did not analyze police officers, they were analyzing duels, but some of the same parallels apply.

Mythbusters did a twenty-four-foot test which ended up with Adam being able to draw and fire his pistol to get shots on his target. They also did a twenty-foot example which gave the same result. Any distance closer than twenty feet meant that Adam would get stabbed every time.

Mythbusters concluded that distances shorter than twenty feet meant that the guy with the knife was always able to stab someone. Keep this in mind... ALWAYS. I am not that good with math, but it always equates to 100% of the time the bad guy wins.

This distance to me is frightening. This means the lady with pepper-spray in her purse had twenty-one feet to prepare and most likely lost seven feet due to inattention.

Discovering Your Trouble Bubble

Once she realizes she is under attack (if she does), Mrs. Pepper Spray is distracted because her one-thousand-dollar phone has to be put away without dropping it and cracking the screen. She then has to find the pepper spray in her purse. Then has to disable the safety and point it in the right direction. She will realistically need about three seconds to get all this done. But she only has about 1.5 seconds from twenty-one feet, and she saw the threat at fifteen feet away instead. This will not turn out well for Mrs. Pepper Spray.

The Mythbusters test and the testing done by Tueller does not include any stress in the situation; it was a stagnant, quasi-scientific benchmark using averages: the average guy, average height, average weight. The people they used were people they knew at the end of the knife blade. The people that were doing the test didn't really want to murder them, hurt them, or subdue them in a real knife battle. The likelihood that you will come out of a knife fight without some damage is not real, even if you are the best-trained gunfighter in the world.

We put this to the test in our own violence lab. When we gave our snarling neanderthals even a minimum reward for clearing the distance in less than 1.5 seconds, we concluded that breaking the 1.5-second mark can be done. Let's just say for the sake of the argument that the reward was steak and beer. If we got a head start and hit the twenty-one-foot mark, we were faster. One and a half seconds is no time at all.

The movies have done fighting, gunshots, and violence an injustice. We think that once we hear the pop or bang of gunfire that the bad guy will magically fly backward and there will be a big explosion. A car will flip over on its side and buildings will crumble. This is simply not true. Fights last less than ten seconds on average. Hitting someone just plain hurts and a gunshot wound is survivable, and when your adrenaline is cranked up, gunshots can feel like a bee sting, so I've been told. I've never been shot.

The fact is that real gun wounds take a while to take effect and the bad guy will keep coming because he still has liquid in him that is leaking through a tiny hole. There is no flying backward when the bullet hits. Keep in mind if you are considering a concealed weapon permit that even though you may fire your weapon at the assailant, he may not actually feel the impact and may not even realize that he is hit because he is so full of adrenaline and or multiple happy pills. He will only stop when he has no more blood pulsing through his veins to keep him conscious, or he is knocked out by a blow to the head.

I know this is morbid. I am just giving you a glimpse of what is real so that you can make good choices and decisions later. Police officers have to make these choices every day when they put on their uniform. You wanted to learn how to think like a cop. This is it.

What really happens when the attacker is yelling, cursing and threatening you?

The answer is that your stress and anxiety will go through the roof. Everything starts to narrow and focus on your threat, which is a natural instinct God has built into your DNA. As you feel your body take over because of this natural fight, flight, or freeze response, you also feel like you are losing control. Your heart starts to beat faster, and you feel like it will beat out of your chest. Your body is doing its job by getting the blood to the vital organs and retracting blood from your non-vital organs. Your fingers don't work or don't feel like they are working as well. Your vision is beginning to blur on the sides like an over-photoshopped selfie on social media. You cannot see a clear avenue of escape to either side of you because the sides of your vision are blurred out. Your hearing becomes muffled and fuzzy, which is called audio exclusion. All of this means that you are not going to react well as a citizen who has not pre-practiced this type of stress inoculation in this reactionary distance known as the twenty-one-foot rule.

Keep in mind that bad guys can also work through the pain of the popular mace or pepper spray that seems to be a security blanket among women. They carry it as a badge of honor in a pink container dangling on a hook on their purse.

Discovering Your Trouble Bubble

The product can be effective. However, they have to realize that they will have to disable the lock, point it in the right direction, hope they don't have a wind blowing in their face, and deploy the fire-breathing squirt gun on a smaller target than a grape from as far as six to twelve feet away, which is the average range of a pepper spray canister. Most women have never tested how long this will take and what the effects are if the wind is going the wrong direction. What if they end up spraying themselves? Now they are blind and vulnerable to the very attack they are trying to prevent. Not good!

As police officers, we have to go through training by being sprayed with pepper spray, the painful tears of the devil. The pain is uncomfortable, but anyone can fight through the pain if they put their minds to it. A villain who is dead set to hurt you and hyped up on happy pills may be able to fight through pepper spray pain to get what he is after. This is something to keep in mind as you build your awareness.

So, what do you do to develop your own personal Trouble Bubble and avoid a violent encounter?

I love teaching about the twenty-one-foot rule and developing your personal Trouble Bubble in my seminars because the distance is eye-opening, if not jaw-dropping. It is impossible to gather all the information needed to do what you want and need to do within twenty-one feet. Even at slower speeds in our own personal, non-threatening violence lab, people start to feel anxious. Even though there is no threat.

Typically, I will take out a measuring tape to find out what a real and accurate twenty-one-foot distance is. I will leave it on the floor so that everyone will know there is no cheating. I will ask for volunteers that carry a firearm, pepper spray, or some tactical device that they feel that they have trained well enough with to launch the device against an attacker.

I or one of our crew will stand at the twenty-one-foot marker of the measuring tape, and the potential victim stands at the other end. If it is a female, it is usually a purse that she has the safety device in. For our purposes, we have a demo purse that she can familiarize herself with and use. She will need to find and deploy this safety device against the attacker that she now knows is coming. As I am talking with them about their device, I cue the attacker to launch. The attacker starts walking aggressively toward the victim without saying a word. Keep in mind that he is walking and not running or yelling as he is running. There is little pressure and little adrenaline pumping through the veins of the victim or the attacker. This is not a real attack yet. There is a realization that something is about to happen, they just don't know what. The average time that it takes the pretend attacker to walk to a potential victim is about three seconds or about

Discovering Your Trouble Bubble

double the time that it would take an aggressive or violent attacker to clear the same distance.

The result is jaw-dropping. They take their eyes off of the attacker to find the tactical safety device. They lose track of time and space. And ninety percent of them freeze in place. Finally, the attacker is right in front of them, reaches out, and touches their shoulder. My usual audience is women. Their eyes are now open to the twenty-one-foot rule and the implications that it could have if they are threatened and or attacked.

Most of them will not even be able to get to their weapon of choice, let alone use it. This demonstration is powerful when you see the lights come on about distances with even a little bit of adrenaline. There seems to be a small bit of adrenaline that kicks in at the tail end of the pretend attacker's walk when he reaches out to touch them. They realize they were not ready. They did not move. They wasted time looking for their safety gadget, then, tag. You're it.

The above example is all done in good fun, and we spend some time in serious laughter, but the example sticks with you for a lifetime. Distance matters.

To put measurements in a different light than a measuring tape: there are two standard garage sizes for a two car garage in America. One standard two car garage is about twenty-four feet by twenty-four feet. The second standard

Discovering Your Trouble Bubble

for a garage is twenty feet by twenty feet. If you don't have a tape measure handy, go out and stand in your garage and imagine that an attacker is coming at you from the far side of the garage and you have to do something within one and a half seconds to save your life.

If you want to get more vivid with the garage experiment, have a family member or good friend charge you at random from across the garage. Again, even though you know you will not be hurt, your adrenaline may increase, and your heart may start pumping out of your chest. Your eyes may focus on just the threat. This is natural, and you should embrace it, knowing that it is put there for a reason and purpose. It is there to protect you and give you focus on your target when you are in danger.

You can develop your own personal twenty-one-foot rule with the Trouble Bubble. The Trouble Bubble does not have to be twenty-one feet as in the above examples. The area includes elements of awareness that we have talked about previously as well as a combination of the twenty-one-foot rule. My personal distance with someone I don't know, and I feel uneasy about, seems to be about twenty-five feet.

Let's say that you are walking in a parking lot and notice someone is acting strange about 100 yards away. You do not have to get within twenty-one feet for your spider senses to kick in, they have just entered your expanded Trouble Bubble, and you can keep an eye on them as you make your

Discovering Your Trouble Bubble

way to your vehicle or through the parking lot. Now if you have to pass this strange person closely to get to your car, then you may want to do things to keep him out of your Trouble Bubble. You may want to leave the area and notify the police or security. You may want to adjust what you are carrying or get a handle on your personal security device ahead of the time you will need it because you know that at twenty-one feet you will only have about one and a half seconds or less to react to a violent attack.

Other things to do to increase your awareness of your own personal space is to get a tape measure and measure out twenty-one feet. You can see how comfortable you are at that distance with a person on the other end walking at you with purpose and vigor. Now increase that distance to where you feel you can raise your hands to protect your vital organs and mount a counterattack if needed. You can also use that distance to practice getting to your personal safety device of choice. Better yet would be to get to your personal safety device and launch an attack with it, so you know your limitations with the device. Good luck finding a volunteer when you are using pepper spray.

My personal Trouble Bubble distance is about twenty-five feet of safety space all around me. My bubble is rather large if you think about a twenty-five-foot distance all around me from the front, sides, and back. My comfort level in talking with a normal stranger that I don't know but I have

Discovering Your Trouble Bubble

determined is not a threat is about ten to fifteen feet. A person who I am comfortable with is about five to six feet, just out of arms reach when you think about it.

When we were talking about the fight, flight, or freeze moment, realize that you do not have to be frozen as a person is walking or running toward you. Practice getting off the target line of the person running at you. Why would you stand there just to get hit? The person cannot change directions fast enough if you just adjust from your spot by a couple of steps to the left or right.

This experiment can be done with the tape measure as well, again, from the twenty-one-foot mark on a tape measure. As someone is running toward you as fast as they can, they will have a hard time changing directions to follow your movement. If you simply step to the side you will increase the time it can take for the bad guy to harm you because they may, in fact, blow right by you in the first place. The bad guy will then have to change directions to come back at you. Practice with a tape measure again at about twenty-one feet. When your fake aggressor runs at you in a straight line at about the ten to fifteen-foot mark, move to the side two or three steps or run to the side if you have room.

Moving and not freezing is hard at first but the more you practice, the more it will become natural and the quicker you will be able to react. Police officers use this technique all

Discovering Your Trouble Bubble

the time in training and on the street. I can still hear my defensive tactics instructor barking, "Step offline!"

As you go through the above steps and pick your awareness points, start to think about distances you will need to develop your personal Trouble Bubble. Your personal space can be honed over time. It can start out as large as you like and shrink over time and practice. This space is your own to do what you will with it. It is your new imaginary self-defense friend. Develop this friendship over time so that when you take The Trouble Bubble out for a walk, he surrounds you with awareness protection.

Discovering Your Trouble Bubble

Developing a Mental Self Defense

Along with physical self-defense and awareness, it is imperative that you develop a mental self-defense that will keep you on track and focused. The more seminars I do, the more I realize that people take my classes for two reasons.

The first reason is that people see what is on the news and in their social media feeds and realize that they are vulnerable and want to be safe. They need a place to start to learn about violence and how to deal with violence the correct way. They may not have the time to do a martial arts class two to three times a week but want recommendations and a place to start. They hear second-hand stories of people who have gone through a violent, traumatic life event and they do not want the next story to be them. They are scared, and they should be. The world is violent and getting worse.

As I type this, I just heard about a media story that broke about a person who was gathering signatures against an online video game manufacturer for a violent video game. I was curious so I listened in to the broadcast. The video game was actually called Active Shooter or something to that effect. The violence in the game depicted school shootings

Developing a Mental Self Defense

where the actor in the game, the person with the controller, was walking into the school and getting points for how many civilians or SWAT officers he or she could kill. This disgusts me! But that is how the world is turning now. Brace yourself!

As of the last editing of this book the manufacturer has taken the game offline. He stated that he does have a right to produce the game and it may land on shelves in the future, but for now, it is out of circulation.

The second type of person who takes my seminars are the ones who have had a violent encounter or close call themselves. They come with good questions and specific situations that they want help dealing with. They are looking for answers to past failings and questions on how to act or react for the future.

In a class on violence and awareness, my answer to both types of people is that if violence is placed in your life and you have no other choice but violence to stay alive… chose violence and stay alive. Sometimes when violence is brought to you, it is the only answer for you and your family to remain safe. Don't sugar coat it. Chose violence if violence lands in your lap. It may be a hard thing to live with afterward, though.

There is another type of violence that is lurking in the darkness waiting to be talked about. This type of violence is how you treat yourself. If you do not give yourself permission to hurt someone else, you will be giving them permission to hurt you.

This is a choice you have made that says, "you have not given yourself permission to love yourself enough to protect yourself." I am giving you permission to love yourself enough to protect yourself and your family because you are worth it.

If you need a personal note from me giving permission, I will gladly provide you with a personal, handwritten note giving you permission to love yourself enough to protect yourself. You are worth it. Get ahold of me and it will happen.

If you acknowledge that you may have trouble finding enough self-worth because of your past or even your current situation, then the following may help. It has helped me forge ahead when I thought things were at an end.

BE GRATEFUL:

Being grateful for even the simple things will help you to realize that things are not as bad as you may have perceived them to be in the first place. Realize that you have a lot going for you if you really take the time to think about it. Even if you start out with the mundane and work your way to the more complex, you have things to be thankful for.

Developing a Mental Self Defense

Have an attitude of gratitude. When you get up in the morning, set time aside to be grateful for something, anything! You will start to lose focus on yourself and gain focus on what it is in the world that is helping you.

I like to make this a morning ritual to really kick-start the day. It is like your daily coffee for survival. So, have a rich cup of Arabica Morning Grateful Blend. You are alive. You're breathing, you are loved, you are nice, you can see enough to read this… be grateful for it. It will change everything.

When I was down on myself, I would get up in the morning and would force myself to write down simple things that made me smile and would carry me through the day. These were the first items on my list when I started: I am grateful for my wife, I am grateful for healthy kids, I am grateful to have legs that work, I am grateful to have a good sense of humor… now be funny! I am not super excited to share my stupid list, but it is what it is. I know it is not earth-shattering, it is just real. That was my list.

I am now grateful that I made the stupid grateful list. I am not much more sophisticated now. I wrote the other day that I was grateful that I am snarky and have a self-deprecating sense of humor. If I can make fun of myself before someone else makes fun of me and actually hurts my delicate feelings, then I am ahead for the day. This is your list, you can hide it wherever you want. It feels great to get it on paper, but you can also just say things out loud on the way to work. I don't always put things to paper, but when I do, it feels so much more solid and powerful.

Sometimes when I get down on myself, I will still take a moment and write a list to force myself to be grateful. I am so grateful for that stupid list! But I still hate that first one.

HAVE A TARGET FOR IMPROVEMENT:

Choose to improve something in your life. Work on your project with curiosity and passion. It can be anything that you have a passion for but have never quite had the gumption to finish or even start. It could be weight loss, public speaking, writing a book, or focused attention on one area of life like relationships. You know what you have always wanted to do. Develop a plan and a target date to achieve your goal. Now, work on it with curiosity and vigor. You will find yourself daydreaming on what you can do, accomplish, and finish rather than dwelling on why you are feeling bad about whatever.

I used simple and achievable targets at first. I chose to lose sixty pounds in five-pound achievable targets and gave them all a date. Did I miss some dates? You bet I did! But I marched forward and was determined to get to where I was going.

I chose to go to Mexico with my wife without the kids. I chose to figure out how to write a book and help people even though I have no idea how to do that. And I still don't, but look at me go!

I chose to put together a woman's self-defense class. I was able to finish all of those things because I put a date on it and told people that I would do it. I promised them and committed to them that it would be finished and done by a specific date.

Imagine that I had promised to take my wife to a beautiful all-inclusive resort in Mexico on a specific date. I gave her my word that I would be ready and able to go. Then, the date came and I was not ready, did not plan for the plane tickets, and did not book the resort. I might be single now. Alas, I am not single and am happily married because I gave myself a goal and a target for travel.

I did the same with my excess weight. My wife Jenny could not lose the weight for me. I promised that I would lose sixty pounds within a time frame or else something bad would happen. I would lose face and lose a bet. The only thing I would not lose if I didn't lose the weight was the weight. It was gone because I said I would, but it was hard. Real hard. I have kept it off because I don't want to go through that again!

HAVE FUN:

Have fun with your life. There is far too much seriousness in life. Turn on the news for half a second and you can't help but run into all the tragedy and heartache. Leave the news off. They can solve their own problems. Use that time to do something fun. Keep it simple, have fun, smile, and laugh. You deserve to take a break from the drama of "self-improvement" and have fun for fun's sake.

I love a good ole belly laugh. The kind of laugh that makes you snort uncontrollably, and you think you may pass out because you are losing air. But as we get older, the trials of life get in the way, and we forget how to laugh. Don't forget! Reach into that lost region and yank out a full handful of belly laughter. Whatever makes you smile, laugh and belly laugh... do that!

I love life and I love golf. Most of the time I am laughing at my golf game, so it is a good combination. They say that laughter is the best medicine, so laugh often and laugh hard, even about the hard things in life.

GIVE YOURSELF PERMISSION:

I gave myself permission to be powerful, to achieve more, do more, live more, have more fun, and stop the self-doubt. But to be honest, this permission didn't completely come from me. Yes, I had to eventually give myself permission. However, the first step came from a mentor that saw a spark in me. He gave me the permission to turn that spark into a blazing inferno. I am giving you that permission. Otherwise, I wouldn't be laboring over this book. I believe in you. Now you believe in you enough to believe you are important enough to protect. Your family is important enough to protect. Take it.

We are told so many times that we need to have permission to do things, but we are unsure of who to ask for it. Ask yourself, but if you need to ask someone else, then ask me. I will tell you that; I am giving you permission to be what you want to be. Be powerful. Feel free to achieve what you have set out to do. Do more with your life. Achieve the success that you have dreamt of. I give you permission to love yourself enough to protect yourself. Live your life with passion. Work toward your dreams and have more fun.

MAKE MISTAKES:

Give yourself permission to make mistakes. Learn and improve from your mistakes. Learn from your failures, laugh about them, and move forward.

The first time I spoke in front of a group of people I lost my notes and I lost a sale that would have fed my family for a month. I lost the respect of the church I was talking to at the time. But I walked next door and nailed the presentation, made the sale, and gained their respect and a friendship for a lifetime. I still did not have the notes that I had lost for my earlier presentation, but I learned how to talk without a PowerPoint and notes as a backup. That failed presentation changed my life because I learned from it and moved on.

Developing a Mental Self Defense

The first time I grappled with someone in the Jiu-Jitsu gym I attended, I was twisted in a pretzel by a girl half my age and a quarter my size. I was embarrassed but learned and improved. I could have quit, but I got curious and passionate about learning. I learned from my mistakes, and now I don't let little girls beat me up anymore.

SHARE WHAT YOU ARE DOING:

Share what you are doing with others. You never know when your success or failures may affect the people around you. Others will use your story to either avoid making your mistakes or learn from your success. Regardless, the act of teaching and sharing will increase your ability to help and train others. Either way, you are helping. So, feel good about yourself, keep going, keep learning, and keep sharing.

EXERCISE HELPS - THE MIND NOT THE BODY

If you look up on YouTube how to exercise you will spend the next few months being confused if not completely frustrated, which will land you right back to the couch. On the couch, you will accomplish very little sit-ups or pushups, and your gym membership is rotting as you catch up on the latest season of the Jersey Shore or whatever your guilty pleasure is. You will not accomplish anything, and you will wake up discouraged, just like yesterday.

Instead, this is my recommendation:

Developing a Mental Self Defense

Join a gym. Plan on going to the gym for at least three months. Give yourself permission to hate the gym after three months. For the first three months, you don't have to love the gym, but you do have to go. Promise me though that you won't love it, just tolerate it, and keep the hate talk to yourself for three months. Also, don't ask for help from Youtube, Facebook, Google, or your annoying friend who is all muscle and only eats chicken breasts and broccoli.

Start at the gym by working up a sweat walking, running, biking, or something aerobic, but sweat a little. You can even watch some cool YouTube videos of people talking on their phones and walking into stuff. Loads of fun! Just don't laugh so hard you fall off the treadmill.

Lift some light things a bunch of times and then lift some heavy things a few times. When you feel your muscles starting to burn, stop. Go take a shower and call it a day. Do it again tomorrow and for the next 90 days. I know you will skip some days. Forgive yourself and keep going. I know you will pick up a doughnut or eat an extra slice of pizza. The gym is not actually for your muscles, it is for your brain. You will focus more, achieve more, and do more if you spend about twenty to thirty minutes of exercising a day. A byproduct of working out is that you will begin to lose the muffin top and you will actually begin to look like how you feel in your head: powerful and focused, ready to take on the world in your own way. You will also become more alert and feel better about yourself. Good for you! You are killing it!

After you have exercised for a while with no plan and want to get complicated, feel free to hire a coach, buy a book, and watch YouTube all you want. Talk to muscle-bound Vinnie who only eats chicken and broccoli. Just don't over complicate your initial action of going to the gym. If you think about it too hard, you are doing something wrong. You can always over complicate things later, for now, keep it simple.

PRAY

This is maybe the scariest thing to do, but once you do, it will change your life for the positive.

It is really simple: talk to God about your life out loud and with passion. Answers will come. I will not promise that your every whim and desire will be answered with a booming voice that says, *"Yes, you will now get what you want."* But what I can promise is that you will feel a sense of ease because a higher power has your back.

Praying will give you stress relief. Speaking your wants, desires, troubles, and your ideas to God will give you a sense that someone else is on your side and willing to help. You can direct all your thoughts to God, he will listen and provide for you, protect you, and assist you in your life.

Developing a Mental Self Defense

Using the tools above, I have given myself permission to write and speak when those things used to scare me. I have also given myself the permission to love myself and help others, which is my passion even though I squashed it for years.

I have stepped out in faith and started speaking more frequently. I hope to be able to travel internationally to teach and train people on how to avoid violence. Using the tools I have talked about and my addiction to helping people, I have refocused my attention on helping civilian businesses share with their workers how to think like police officers, develop a 360 awareness of their surroundings, and use mental self-defense methods to keep themselves and their families safe.

Bonus:
Top Strategies When Faced with Physical Violence

People ask my opinion all the time. The question usually starts out with "What would you do if...?" Or ,"I was in this or that situation, what would have you done?"

This opinion gathering always feels a little like a trap to me, but I have a few rules that I follow. The rules can go fast or slow depending on the situation. I have seen a situation go from nothing to full speed violence even though the strategies were followed. At least the strategies were attempted. Also, in the strategies you will notice there is a contingency for violence.

DON'T BE THERE:

The number one strategy for not being involved in violence is to not be there. This seems simple because sometimes life places violence in your lap and you have to deal with it. But, what if you DID have a choice?

I consider it a choice to go to a bar that I know over-serves alcohol to a clientele of degenerates. Why would I

Bonus: Top Strategies When Faced with Physical Violence

choose that? I wouldn't. Why would I walk down an alley that smells like a men's urinal for a ten-step shortcut when I could walk on Main Street USA with witnesses and people? I would not do that. It is called being smart and keeping your awareness on point.

In both choices, can violence happen even if you make the best choices ever? Yes, they can, and yes, they do! They are just less likely. Hedge your bets, as they say.

NEVER ESCALATE:

Why would someone escalate a fight or episode of violence when there is no need? De-escalate and be safe. However, I would suggest that it is better for you to walk away with some hurt feelings than get a ride in an ambulance and own a hospital bill.

It can take just two hits for you to be scared or incapacitated for life. The first hit may be a lucky one driven in by an attacker when it connects with your temple causing you to stumble and fall unconscious before you hit the ground. The second hit is the jagged-edged curb to the sidewalk that your head connects with, causing permanent damage to your moneymaker. You end up with a two hundred and fifty-nine thousand reconstruction bill for your face so that you don't have to breathe through a tube, all because you threw your hands out to the sides of your body, puffed out your chest, and said, "Bring it!" That was a bad decision and avoidable.

It may be better to say, "you win," put your hands in front of you, and walk away. I am just suggesting that is a better choice if you have that choice to make.

GIVE THEM A CHOICE:

When you are faced with a violent decision where you have a choice, the choice is always better to walk away than it is to stay and fight. Usually, if the other party is still talking and puffing out his chest, the fight is avoidable. If they really wanted a fight or to bring violence to a situation, then it would have already happened. They are looking for a way out. Give them an easy way out, if possible.

You can give them the same opportunity with simple de-escalation statements that we have talked about in this book. Such as, "You win!" which is my favorite.

If "you win," is not in the cards, give the aggressor a choice such as: "You don't want a part of this, it would be better to walk away." Or, "Listen, you will end up in the hospital and then jail if you continue," or "You can leave, the choice is yours," or, "I don't want a part of this, I am leaving."

HANDS UP:

By having your hands up, you create a barrier that is hard to get around. The attacker will have to find a way to break the barrier to get inside your hands and arms to something

Bonus: Top Strategies When Faced with Physical Violence

that can hurt you. By doing this, he may choose to leave you alone. You may even look like you know what you are doing.

If he does not choose to leave you alone, you will have your natural black belt defenses in place and ready for action. Split seconds matter.

Do not close your fists like you are in a boxing match. Do the opposite of what you see on television. Splay your fingers wide open and just talk with your hands out in front of your chest. This looks natural and does not invite a fight.

If a fight or violence lands in your lap, you already have your natural protectors up and are ready.

POWER OVER TECHNIQUE:

If you do not have any technique and have not taken a self-defense class or have a punching bag or kicking bag for practice, keep in mind brute force and power. Strike through the target. I am not talking about striking through a piece of paper, I am talking about being able to knock your aggressor to the ground with your punch, kick, tackle, or throw. Whatever you do, do it with as much force and vigor as you can muster.

Martial artists all over the world are silently screaming at me while mentally gouging my eyes with ninja stars from their crisscross-applesauce seated positions in their empty dojo's. (This is what I imagine they do when they are not teaching a class). Don't get me wrong. I believe in

Bonus: Top Strategies When Faced with Physical Violence

technique. I believe in learning a martial art and self-defense to protect yourself. In fact, I would highly recommend Brazilian Jiu-Jitsu and Krav Maga. I believe that you will be better off and safer if you have a technique to back your power. However, if you don't have any training or experience, then you better bring the power and ferocity of a momma bear protecting her cubs.

You should have already hit something with the same power and ferocity that you will hit a bad guy with or you won't know how to do it. If you give them a love tap in order not to hurt them, they may take your life. Own that and obliterate your attacker.

Without technique and practice, you may miss your target. You may hurt yourself before you put down your aggressor. But make no mistake about power. If you hit someone with full force and power going through your target, through the body, through the head, through the groin, you WILL do damage. Even if you miss the mark by a small margin, you are creating time for an escape or another strike if needed. By using power to create distance, you may be able to get away while the attacker is catching his breath from the beating he just received. He may even think twice about re-attacking, knowing you are a hard target.

Brute force and power is no guarantee that you will evade injury, but if you do not have technique, use power to survive and fight for your life.

Bonus: Top Strategies When Faced with Physical Violence

A saying that I use sometimes because of its powerful visual is:
"Fight like you are the third monkey trying to get on Noah's Ark!"

This creates a visual in your mind's eye of a monkey going crazy in a fight for his life and the survival of his gene pool. He will do anything to get on that boat. You should do anything to survive in a fight for your life. Do not play patty cake with someone who is trying to hurt you. Do not give up. Do not slack off. Be brutal. Be forceful. Be powerful. Do not let up until the danger is gone.

MANTRA:
When you are preparing your mind for the fight you may never have to get into, remember that you may need to use violence to get out of a violent attack. I hope you never have to use violence in this way but, if you have to, you are giving yourself permission for protecting yourself and your family.

Things to remember:

"If they can't breathe, they can't fight; if they can't see, they can't fight; if they can't function, they can't fight; and if they can't think, they can't fight."

Bonus: Top Strategies When Faced with Physical Violence

If they can't breathe, they can't fight:

If your attacker is gasping for air, they cannot chase you, and they cannot fight. Your targets should be the solar plexus, throat, and groin.

If they can't see, they can't fight:

If your attacker cannot see because he has an eye poked, severely scratched, or popped, then he will lose concentration on you, and he will only be able to think about the pain. You can get away.

If they can't function they can't fight:

When your attacker does not have functioning body parts, he will not be able to chase you. If his knee is out of joint or broken, he will not be able to physically chase you. If his arm is broken, he will not be able to grab you. It will be physically impossible for them to catch you as you are getting away from the situation. If you were to break the eardrum, your attacker would not be able to walk straight because his equilibrium would be out of whack. He couldn't stand straight or he would throw up, let alone chase you.

If they can't think, they can't fight.

If your attacker cannot think he will not be able to carry out his plans. He will lose concentration on you and will only be able to concentrate on pain or staying conscious. If you strike a person in the groin hard enough, with full force,

Bonus: Top Strategies When Faced with Physical Violence

either male or female, that person would not be able to think or breathe, and you will be able to get away safely.

Conclusion

As a police officer, at times myself and other officers are thrust into violent situations. This is not our choice for the most part. If we had a choice, the majority of us would choose to end it peacefully, as I hope you will. We have taken an oath to help the people of our communities. Experience has shown us that violence is a part of our world now, and violence may be unavoidable.

I want you to have an educated choice about being a victim. Choose to protect you and your family. You are important.

Stay safe.

Conclusion

About the Author

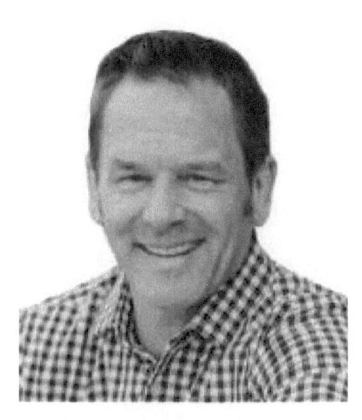

Josh Mercer is an experienced Police Officer who delivers powerful workshops, seminars and keynotes that give you the tools you need if you are involved in an unexpected situation. Josh sees violence daily on the job and is driven to prevent it. Because of his experience with law enforcement, Josh has a passion to help others. He takes pride in providing the best personalized service possible. Josh has an extraordinary commitment that he calls "an addiction" to helping people. He has fostered this desire into a talent for helping people to learn how to stay safe prior to needing police services. Josh teaches people how to think "like police officers" in his workshops and seminars. He teaches proven techniques to people just like you, that can be used immediately. You will go home from one of his workshops knowing that you have the upper hand in a violent situation and you will learn how you can proactively deter most violent situations from happening before they happen.

Josh works with civilian companies taking the blindfold off violence; empowering people to be safe and live empowering lives. You can find out more about Josh Mercer or learn how to book him for your event on his website: **www.thinklikeacopseminars.com**

Think like a Cop

Think like a Cop

Think like a Cop

Disclaimer & Copyright Information

The information contained in this book is not to be considered advice for guaranteed strategies, nor is the content intended to offer phycological advice, full prevention, or guaranteed outcomes, nor is it a substitute for calling on medical professionals for help, or professional law enforcement for assistance during times of criminal activity or other. Please consult your local law enforcement agency for any matter(s) affecting you or your personal safety. Contact an attorney for crimes you believe have been committed against you, contact a professional counselor or seek professional help if you need other assistance.

Some of the events, locales, and conversations have been recreated from memories. In order to maintain their anonymity, in some instances, the names of individuals and places have been changed. As such, some identifying characteristics and details may have changed. All content is original, and any similar instances should be considered a coincidence.

Although the author and publisher have made every effort to ensure that the information in this book was correct at press time, the author and publisher do not assume and hereby disclaim any liability to any party for any loss, damage, or disruption caused by errors or omissions, whether such errors or omissions result from negligence, accident, or any other cause.

All quotes, unless otherwise noted,
are attributed to Josh Mercer.

Cover illustration, book design, and production
Copyright © 2019 by Tribute Publishing LLC
www.TributePublishing.com

www.ingramcontent.com/pod-product-compliance
Lightning Source LLC
Chambersburg PA
CBHW030326080526
44584CB00012B/731